Published in association with MacGregor and Luedeke Literary, Inc.

Cover design by Studio Gearbox

Cover photo © 895Studio, le adhiz, TairA, antart, Henry Hazboun / Shutterstock

Interior design by Chad Dougherty

For bulk, special sales, or ministry purchases, please call 1-800-547-8979. Email: Customerservice@hhpbooks.com

M This logo is a federally registered trademark of the Hawkins Children's LLC. Harvest House Publishers, Inc., is the exclusive licensee of this trademark.

ONE-MINUTE PRAYERS is a registered trademark of The Hawkins Children's LLC. Harvest House Publishers, Inc., is the exclusive licensee of the federally registered trademark ONE-MINUTE PRAYERS.

One-Minute Prayers® for Women with Cancer
Copyright © 2022 by Niki Hardy
Published by Harvest House Publishers
Eugene, Oregon 97408
www.harvesthousepublishers.com

ISBN 978-0-7369-8391-4 (hardcover)
ISBN 978-0-7369-8392-1 (eBook)

Printed in China

23 24 25 26 27 28 29 30 / RDS / 10 9 8 7 6 5 4 3

Contents

You're Not Alone in This

The doctor sighed heavily. The tumor they'd found was either cancer or lymphoma, yet I hardly flinched at the news.

"Oh, is there a third option?" I asked calmly.

Maybe it was denial. Maybe it was the anesthesia drugs still coursing through my veins, fogging my brain. Or perhaps the Lord's peace descended just when I needed it. Regardless, I didn't break down. Not then.

Your tears may have flowed immediately, the what-ifs of your midnight worry sessions suddenly morphing into reality. Or maybe you slowly folded into yourself like a deflating bouncy castle. Perhaps you gasped, your hand racing to stifle the eruption of a primeval wail, before gathering yourself to pepper your doctor with a million questions. Or maybe your diagnosis was so unexpected you simply sat, dazed and stunned in shocked silence.

However you reacted—and please know there's no right or wrong way—you're here because you have cancer, and for that I'm so sorry. It stinks. It just does.

More than anything, I want you to know you're not alone. No matter what cancer chucks your way, I want to journey through this with you, my hand on your shoulder, as we allow God to be our daily companion through these Scriptures, prayers, and words of encouragement.

I know the fear, worry, overwhelm, confusion, and yes, even anger, is very real, so I've been praying for you as I write. Your cancer's probably overshadowing everything right now, but I want you to know something: You've got this. How am I so sure? Because I know God's got you.

My diagnosis came a mere six weeks after I lost my sister to cancer—and just six years after I lost my mom. Still grieving, I felt like it was my turn. So I understand. I fought through chemo, radiation, surgery, more chemo, and enough scans and blood work to keep a fully staffed lab in overtime. As I fought, I needed to hear a few key things every day, sometimes every minute. Now I want to pass them on to you, my friend.

First, though it might seem obvious, I want to make sure you hear this: God is good, and he likes you, and he's 100 percent for you 100 percent of the time. When cancer rips our world apart, it's easy to think he's mad or punishing us, but that simply isn't true. If we fully understood the enormity of his love, it would blow our minds. So remember, you are loved—passionately and unconditionally.

Second, God hasn't left you. He isn't off helping someone more "deserving," like the missionary couple you support in Thailand, or Janice at church who leads Bible studies and didn't sleep around in college. Regardless of whether you can see him, feel him, or hear him, God is with you and isn't going anywhere. Saint Augustine's testimony is true for you too: "God is nearer to me than I am to myself."[1]

Last, please don't get in a tizzy about the hows, whens, wheres and whats of prayer. We tend to think "proper" prayers are eloquent, bursting with scriptural references, and uttered in profound faith. But this is a myth. Yes, those prayers are great, but don't let your relationship with God be held back by your humanity: the fear of not praying perfectly, the inability to pray more than a sentence, or the need to simply scream and question God. God's ear is always bent toward us, and the only wasted or "wrong" prayer is the one we don't pray. So my encouragement is to keep it simple, keep it real, and keep it going,[2] which is exactly what I'm here to help you do.

I'm sure you've got teams of professionals steering you through the medical maze of cancer, and I hope you have a tribe of trusted friends bringing meals, running kids to practice, and maybe even throwing laundry in the wash. Perhaps a few close friends and a church community have even committed to praying for you. That's wonderful. No matter how pulled together we normally are, we all need people around us when our world falls apart. God is a God of community, three in one, and because we are built in his image, we are wired for community. My prayer is that through this book I too become part of your tribe.

I've purposefully structured these prayers into easily navigable sections so you can find what you need when you need it most. Feel free to pick and choose, dip and dive, and even hang out in one section for as long as you like. These devotions are for you, and there's no right or wrong way to use them. Scribble in the spaces, read the prayers out loud, or change up my words to make them your own. Do whatever you need so talking to God becomes easier. The important thing is that you invite God in, however that works best for you, even if you're not sure he's there. He knows what you're going through and longs to walk through this with you.

If cancer taught me anything, it's that life doesn't have to be pain-free to be full. I pray this little book helps you discover that too.

When You're Feeling...
Afraid

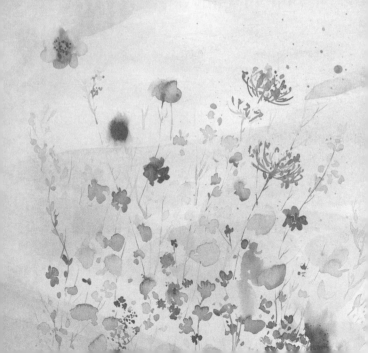

May your *love* always
outshine my darkest fear.

Meeting Fear Head-On

*Do not be anxious about anything, but in every situation,
by prayer and petition, with thanksgiving, present your
requests to God. And the peace of God, which
transcends all understanding, will guard your
hearts and your minds in Christ Jesus.*

PHILIPPIANS 4:6-7

If only God would wave his mighty hand and banish our fear forever. How strong and courageous we'd be! God doesn't want us to feel afraid, but when we do, more than anything he wants us to come to him in the midst of it. He doesn't stop fear's stampede. But he does provide all we need to meet it head-on: prayer, petition, and thanksgiving. Here, knee-deep in our relationship with God, is where we find the peace that guards our hearts.

O Lord, I wish you'd just take my fear away! But I confess, if you did, I'd probably not come to you as much. So in my fear I return to you in prayer—worshipping and praising you, giving thanks for who you are, for what you've done and all you will do. I cry out for all I need. You promise to guard my heart with your peace, and today I need it, Lord. Surround and protect my fragile, fearful heart.

He Is with You

*Be strong and courageous. Do not be afraid or terrified
because of them, for the LORD your God goes with you;
he will never leave you nor forsake you.*

DEUTERONOMY 31:6

Unfortunately, fear isn't something we can simply decide to ignore or shed absentmindedly like a sweater on a warm summer's day. It follows us around unbidden.

On the verge of finally entering the Promised Land, the Israelites were paralyzed by the size of the enemies they faced. God told them to be strong and courageous, and he says the same to you as you face cancer. You too can be strong and courageous. You too can rise above fear and terror. Why? Because just as God was with the Israelites, he is with you, and he will never leave.

Lord God, I'm scared. Really scared. I can't shake the fear overwhelming me, confronting me at every appointment, scan, treatment, and conversation. It keeps me awake and overtakes me. Lord, thank you for being with me. Thank you for never leaving me, ever. Because of your presence, I don't need to be afraid. Today, Lord, whatever cancer enemy I face, remind me of your continued presence. Give me your courage and strength to face it head-on, with you.

Leave Your Fears with God

Cast all your anxiety on him because he cares for you.

1 PETER 5:7

If you're anything like me, you tell God your worries. You probably even try to give them to him. But sooner or later you snatch them back and begin turning them over in your mind—repeatedly, relentlessly. A fisherman casts his fly into a flowing stream and reels it in again and again and again, but God tells us to cast our fears on him once and for all. To leave them with him and walk away. How? In the strength of his love and care. So let's throw our anxiety on him today and then turn and walk away, confident he loves us deeply.

Lord, I know I'm not great at telling you my fears, and the worst at leaving them with you before sneaking back to pick them up. Forgive me. It shows I rank my ability to take care of things higher than yours. I'm sorry. I trust your love. I know you care about everything that keeps me awake at night. Today, as I choose to give it all to you and walk away in the strength of your love and care, may I know your perfect peace.

Stop Spinning

The LORD will fight for you; you need only to be still.

EXODUS 14:14

Moses and the Israelites were camped on the banks of the Red Sea, the Egyptian army bearing down on them. There was nowhere to go, nowhere to hide. In their fear they mumbled and complained. Surely all was lost? When they cried out to God, he didn't tell them to run, fight, or even hide. He simply said, "Be still." He wanted them to keep silent and to be calm. When we stop spinning anxiously in fear-fueled circles, silence our complaining, lay aside our plans of attack, and sit calmly in his presence, he fights for us. What a wonderful thought.

Lord, forgive my anxiety and complaining. It's so much easier to worry, grumble, and fret through a hundred different what-if scenarios than to sit still in your presence. My fears shout louder than your still, small voice—I feel so helpless. And I confess, worrying can feel more productive than sitting still, even in your presence. But with you, all is not lost. Lord, calm my fears. Meet me in the stillness. Fight for me.

Holding You Steady

Do not fear, for I am with you; do not be dismayed,
for I am your God. I will strengthen you and help you;
I will uphold you with my righteous right hand.

ISAIAH 41:10

A tiny babbling stream eventually erodes its way through soil and rock to become a mighty, roaring river. In the same way, ever-present niggling fears wear their way into highways of panic. When we live with this continual fear, it's easy to become disillusioned with God. It's easy to lose hope. Once again, we find the Israelites felt as we do today: exiled and downtrodden, afraid and dismayed. Yet God told them not to. God told them he would strengthen them, help them, and hold them steady. The same is true for you. Can you let God strengthen you? Can you let him help and uphold you?

Fear is my constant companion, one that I can't shake. It's worn me down. Lord, I feel weak, alone, and so afraid. You encouraged the Israelites in exile and told you'd strengthen them, uphold them, and help them. I need that today, Father. In my fear and distress, hold me tight. Don't let me go. Help me, and strengthen me in my weakness. It all feels too much, but you are my God, and you can lift me up.

Your True Shepherd

Even though I walk through the darkest valley,
I will fear no evil, for you are with me;
your rod and your staff, they comfort me.

PSALM 23:4

The valley of cancer is long, dark, and cold. What's ahead is unknown, and every turn in the road sends our minds spiraling.

Somehow, in his darkest place, David could say he feared no evil. His love of God and his years as a shepherd—fighting off wolves with his staff and guiding his sheep along rocky paths—taught him his true Shepherd was with him and would do the same for him. God would be his comfort in the valley. So too, with his rod and staff, the Lord is with you. He will be your abiding comfort.

Lord, this cancer valley has me sick with worry. I wish I could see a way out, but the path is too long, too dark. I'm grateful you're with me and that I'm not alone. Lord, protect me. Wield your rod against everything advancing against me. Guide me with your staff. I don't want to stray from your path or away from you. Let me feel your comfort, Lord. Let me know your guiding presence.

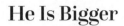

He Is Bigger

Mightier than the thunder of the great waters,
mightier than the breakers of the sea—
the LORD on high is mighty.

PSALM 93:4

If you've ever been on or near the ocean during a storm, you know how it feels to be dwarfed by its unstoppable strength and power. Just as the uncontrollable, raging seas brought fear and anxiety to the Israelites, the crashing waves of cancer leave us weak, afraid, and feeling utterly helpless. The Israelites found peace knowing that despite appearances, their God was mightier than even the most tempestuous seas. We can find that same peace today. Remember, your God is bigger than cancer!

Lord, in the face of cancer, I feel small, powerless, and afraid. But today I look to you. You are stronger, mightier, more powerful. You are the place I find peace. Jesus, just as you calmed the storm for the disciples, would you calm the storm raging in me? Each time the waters of cancer begin to rise, help me focus on you, on all you've done and all you can do and all you will do. Help me walk in your peace. You are mightier than cancer!

When You're Feeling...

Alone

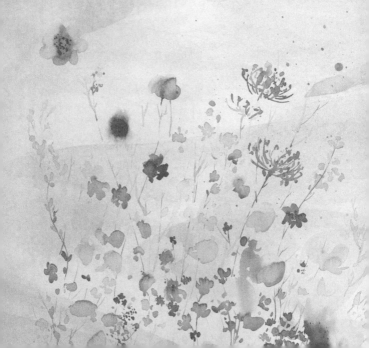

May his love remind me I'm

never alone.

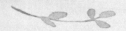

In His Mighty Hand

I am the LORD your God who takes hold of your
right hand and says to you, Do not fear; I will help you.

ISAIAH 41:13

The bad news is only you can walk your cancer journey. No one can sit in the chemo chair, undergo surgery, or fight for you. So no matter how wonderful your friends and family are, battling cancer can be lonely. The good news is you're not alone. God takes your frail, nervous hand in his strong and mighty one, reassuring you of his constant presence and help. What a comfort!

Lord, my friends and family are great, but it's hard for them to understand. Even in the noise and chaos of my people-filled life, I still feel alone. Help me, Lord. Take my hand and hold it tight. Never let me go. You are the Lord my God. With my hand safely in yours, I am secure in the knowledge you'll help me through this. Truly, I need not fear, for with you I'm never alone. Thank you for your hand firmly clasping mine. In my loneliest moments, help me feel your strength and comfort in your steady grasp.

He Knows

*My God will meet all your needs according to
the riches of his glory in Christ Jesus.*

PHILIPPIANS 4:19

Sometimes all we need is a hug, someone to say, "I get it, I've been there," or a friend to pick up our prescriptions. Other times, our loneliness overwhelms us and our solitude is paralyzing.

If that's you today, Paul's reminder to the church in Philippi is for you too. The Lord knows what you need before you do, and he promises to liberally supply everything you need. What a pledge! Today, how can you trust him to meet you in your aloneness and generously provide all your needs?

You know where and how I need help at home, financially, with the kids, and with healing. You're not blind to my ache for understanding or my desire to be seen in my pain. Lord God, meet me in my place of greatest needs. Even though I can't see when or how you'll do it, please take care of those needs. May I never feel alone. Thank you for meeting me in those deepest places. I trust your generosity and presence.

Loved in Your Aloneness

Turn to me and be gracious to me,
for I am lonely and afflicted.

PSALM 25:16

For some reason, it's more acceptable to say we have cancer than to confess we're lonely. When we do admit to feeling alone, people often offer optimistic observations of how our lives are full of people who love us, not understanding that has little to do with it. But where does that leave us? Feeling ashamed of our loneliness, afraid to speak up again, holding our aloneness even closer. Thanks to the psalmist's honesty, we know it's more than okay to cry out to God when we feel this way. Even when no one else offers us grace, God always does. Be encouraged, my friend, and confidently share your loneliness with him, knowing you are totally loved.

I feel so alone in my cancer, Lord. I'm nervous about sharing how I truly feel. I fear their blind optimism, platitudes, and pity. Thank you for your grace and understanding. In my loneliness, turn to me, Lord. Lift the weight of shame and guilt weighing down my weary soul. In my place of deepest need, be gracious to me. In my emptiness, fill me up.

By Your Side

*At my first defense, no one came to my support, but
everyone deserted me. May it not be held against them.
But the Lord stood at my side and gave me strength.*

2 TIMOTHY 4:16-17

You don't have to have cancer long before you hear well-meaning clichés, awkward accounts of someone's uncle dying of the same thing, or the latest seaweed miracle cure. Then, after an influx of meal deliveries and offers of help, there's often silence, as other people's lives move on or they simply struggle to offer ongoing love and support. If you feel deserted, I'm so sorry. Thankfully, God will never leave you. He's in it with you for the long haul. He stands by you, literally at your side, strengthening you.

Lord, it's hard when people don't understand or, feeling awkward and tongue-tied, blurt out something hurtful. It hurts when they simply stop showing up. Help me not to hold it against them. Instead, may I focus on you by my side, strengthening me daily. With you next to me, I have the love and courage to face the day and ask for help when I need it. You will never desert me. You are my strength.

Unwavering Confidence

*A time is coming and in fact has come
when you will be scattered, each to your
own home. You will leave me all alone. Yet
I am not alone, for my Father is with me.*

JOHN 16:32

Unless he was praying alone, Jesus spent his ministry constantly surrounded by people. Then they scattered. He knew they'd leave him to face his trial and crucifixion alone, but confident in his Father's presence, he also knew he'd never be alone. Remember, Jesus knows what it's like to be alone, deserted, and misunderstood. He understands your loneliness. Jesus could endure the horrific journey to the cross thanks to his unwavering confidence in his Father's presence. We can endure anything our cancer journey holds, confident our Father is with us too.

O Jesus, I'm so grateful you know what it feels like to be alone and misunderstood. You too have felt the pain of loneliness. You understand. Lord, strengthen my confidence in your presence. When I doubt it, remind me. In the lonely quiet of my aching heart, whisper your nearness and quench my longing. With you I can endure anything.

Through the Fire

*He said, "Look! I see four men walking
around in the fire, unbound and unharmed,
and the fourth looks like a son of the gods."*

DANIEL 3:25

We might not have chosen to walk through the fire of cancer as a stand against an idolatrous king. But that doesn't make the flames any less terrifying. As Shadrach, Meshach, and Abednego stepped into the furnace, they didn't know if God would deliver them. And as we step into surgery or lie on the scanner, neither do we. However, just like them, we do know an important truth: He's promised to never leave us. We too can trust he's present as we walk through the fire. Let's look for him in the flames of our cancer today.

Lord, you promise to never leave me, but today, as the fires of my cancer rage around me, I feel more alone than ever. Remind me of your presence in the heat of the furnace. Reassure me that you're with me, even if I can't see you or feel your presence. As I go through my day and the flames threaten to engulf me, may I feel your nearness. May I rest in your comfort and protection.

Day and Night

Because of your great compassion you did not abandon them in the wilderness. By day the pillar of cloud did not fail to guide them on their path, nor the pillar of fire by night to shine on the way they were to take.

NEHEMIAH 9:19

Journeying through cancer can feel like wandering through the desert—alone, exhausted, hurting, and confused. The dry, parched land seems endless. The lush, fruitful valley of our precancer days seems distant. Yet the scorching heat can't evaporate God's love. His great compassion shines down, and he never abandons us to wander aimlessly or to fend for ourselves. His presence, his guidance, and his provision are always with us, by day and by night. We simply need to look. Can you see it?

Lord, as I struggle onward in this arid desert, I get more lost, alone, exhausted, and afraid. I'm clinging to the truth that no matter how abandoned I may feel, I'm not forsaken. Your compassion and love have never left. They will never leave. Thank you, Lord. Help me see your presence by day and by night, and show me the way to go. Shine your light on my path.

When You're Feeling...
Sad

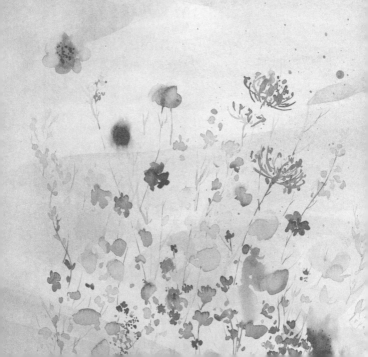

In my sadness, may your *comfort* and *peace* envelop me.

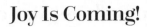

Joy Is Coming!

Weeping may stay for the night,
but rejoicing comes in the morning.

PSALM 30:5

When the day has been rough and we finally slump into bed, it's not just the night's darkness that closes in. All too often we find ourselves spiraling downward emotionally and spiritually as the shadows of sadness and worry envelop us. Comfort, peace, and joy seem agonizingly out of reach. But they're not. Yes, we may weep through the night, but a shout of joy is always waiting as day breaks. Take heart, my friend: Joy is coming! Let your sadness give way to laughter.

Night is the hardest time, Lord. The darkness stretches out endlessly. Tears flow, and life feels drained of joy. You tell me "the nights of crying your eyes out give way to days of laughter,"³ but it doesn't always seem that way. As the glimmer of land on the horizon brings hope and comfort to a sailor lost at sea, may your promise of rejoicing in the morning hold me fast through the darkest nights. With you, joy is always coming. So I give you thanks and praise, even as my pillow dampens with tears.

Your Sadness Matters

Record my misery; list my tears on your scroll—
are they not in your record?

PSALM 56:8

Tears, grief, sadness, and misery—they come free of charge with every diagnosis. And cancer rips the joy out of life faster than you can say, "Do I need chemo?" Honestly, it can all feel so heavy, so endless. Thankfully, God not only sees our sadness but deems it so important that he writes it on his scroll. He even collects each precious tear in his bottle.[4] In your lowest moments, imagine him bottling each one of your tears: You are seen, and you are so very loved. What matters to you matters to God. He forgets neither you nor your tears.

Lord God, whenever I feel low and lost, may the picture of you writing my pain in your book and collecting my tears bring me comfort, hope, and healing. Thank you for the tenderness and love this image brings to mind. The thought of my sadness and grief mattering that much to you revives my wounded and weary heart. It helps me tiptoe through the broken pieces of my life with new strength.

Permission to Weep

Jesus wept.

JOHN 11:35

Stop crying. Buck up. Pull yourself together. Be grateful and look on the bright side. How often have you told yourself something along these lines? If you're anything like me, probably far too frequently. To women who are usually strong, capable, and prepared, tears and sadness can feel weak or self-indulgent. Yet God gave us tear ducts and emotions that can't help but overflow. He gave them to Jesus as well. In his grief and sadness, Jesus wept—without shame and certainly not in weakness. Dear friend, Jesus understands and has led the way. Let's give ourselves permission to be sad, to grieve and weep. It's okay.

Why do I hate crying and feeling sad, Lord, when you created emotions and tears? Forgive me for holding them in when not even Jesus did that. I'm so grateful you understand the ache of grief and sadness and would never tell me to hold it together or get a grip. When I resist my tears, may I remember your leading and example. In my sadness, may I feel your presence and let my tears flow.

Every Single Tear

The Sovereign LORD will wipe away
the tears from all faces.

ISAIAH 25:8

As kids, when we fell and scraped our knees, our moms scooped us up, held us close, tenderly wiped our tears, and reassured us we'd be okay. Cancer is certainly more than a scraped and bloody knee. But no matter how bruised and battered it leaves us, we always have this reassurance, hope, and comfort: One day, Jesus will personally wipe away all our tears. Just as our mothers did when we were kids, our Father in heaven does now. He reminds us, gently, that we'll be okay. He sees today's tears and, in his sovereign love, promises to wipe away every single one.

Lord, I confess, in my pain it's easy to believe you don't see my tearstained face, my grief, my sadness—or, if you do, that they simply don't matter. Quite honestly, I wish you'd wipe them away today, right now, and take this cancer with them. Until you do, Lord, bring me comfort. Reassure me I'm seen and loved and, no matter what, that it will be okay. Hold me tight. Don't let me go. And as I cry my way through whatever's next, remind me of your love.

Your Joy-Filled Harvest

*Those who go out weeping, carrying seed to sow, will
return with songs of joy, carrying sheaves with them.*

PSALM 126:6

Sadness curls us into a ball, beckons us under the
duvet, and tells us to simply forget life for a while.
We promise ourselves we'll get back on track and pick
up our relationship with Jesus when we feel better and
more up to it. Unfortunately, that's not how it works.
No matter how low or lethargic we feel, we're called
to keep sowing seeds by meeting with Jesus and loving those around us. As we do, we're promised a harvest—one so full of joy we burst into song!

*Lord, I want to stop the world and hide away until I feel
happier and more motivated. But I choose to come to you
in my weeping. Help me sow your seeds of love, even if
I scatter them through tears of grief and sadness. Now,
more than ever, I need the fruit of your love, Lord. Grow
your fruit in me: your love, joy, peace, patience, kindness,
goodness, faithfulness, gentleness, and self-control. Then
may it overflow to those around me.*

Top of His List

Blessed are the poor in spirit, for theirs is the kingdom of heaven. Blessed are those who mourn, for they will be comforted.

MATTHEW 5:3-4

If it feels like your cancer has demoted you to the bottom of God's "who's loved and important" list, I understand. Isn't he more interested in people on fire for him, the ones proclaiming the gospel from rooftops and bringing justice and love to the oppressed? Nope, not at all. He calls you—yes, *you*—blessed! Not only that, but in his compassion, he promises comfort. Everyone is at the top of his list. Come to him today and you'll find the comfort you crave.

Lord God, I'm so grateful for these words of Jesus. Remind me how, rather than being forgotten, I'm blessed. My spirit is weak, my heart aches, and I don't feel blessed. Yet even here, in the depths of my sadness, you promise comfort and tell me the kingdom of heaven is mine. Thank you. Your words lift my spirits and bring me hope. As I come to you today with all my sadness on display, put your arms around me so I might know the truth of your promise. Comfort me, Lord.

Puzzle Peace

For God is not a God of disorder but of peace.

1 CORINTHIANS 14:33

Cancer shakes up our lives. Like a completed puzzle that's been returned to its box only to be shaken violently, we're left in unrelenting chaos. Our neatly ordered emotions are left tangled and confused. So it's good to be reminded that our God is not a God of disorder but of peace. No matter how "disordered" your life is today, the God of peace is still with you and for you. May he share that peace and fill you with it, no matter how chaotic and confusing your circumstances continue to be.

I don't like chaos and disorder, Lord. It makes me feel out of control and highlights everything that robs me of joy. Bring your order and peace into my confusion and sadness. Help me navigate through the chaos with a calmness and clarity only you can give. And no matter what my day holds, may I walk in your peace.

When You're Feeling...

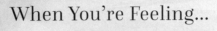
Hurt

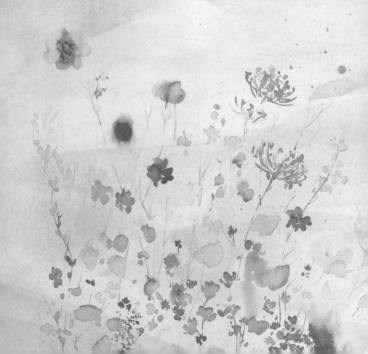

In my pain, may I always turn toward *you*, never away.

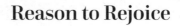

Reason to Rejoice

*In all this you greatly rejoice, though now for a little while
you may have had to suffer grief in all kinds of trials.*

1 PETER 1:6

Hurt makes us hunker down and laser focus on the here and now. Pain consumes our thoughts, its tentacles spreading through every moment, and we wonder, *Why should we rejoice when joy has all but vanished?* Peter, flawed and intimately acquainted with pain, tells us. We rejoice because our hurt is set against the backdrop of our birth into a living hope—an imperishable, unfading, unspoiled, and eternal inheritance—and in it we are guarded by God's power.

Now that's a reason to rejoice!

Lord, like a tidal wave, my pain engulfs me. I'm drowning and it's all I can focus on. Rejoicing is the last thing I feel like doing. Forgive me. In this darkness, let your light—the light of my eternal, living hope in you—pierce through. Fix my eyes on it and help me give thanks and rejoice. You went to the cross to give me that hope, both in my pain and eternally with you. Thank you. Your love sustained you through your suffering and allows me to rejoice in mine.

Saved in Our Shattering

The LORD is close to the brokenhearted
and saves those who are crushed in spirit.

PSALM 34:18

When our hearts break and our spirits are crushed a little more each day, God can seem far away, even uncaring. We lie motionless as we're slid into the scanner, fidget nervously as our oncologist explains test results, or watch the hope fade in our kids' eyes at the news the cancer has returned—and our hearts shatter. Our spirits collapse under the weight of hurt. Yet, even here, "closer is He than breathing, and nearer than hands and feet,"[5] and he saves us in our shattering. Can I encourage you to invite him closer still?

Lord, if I'm honest—and I know I can be with you—I'm fed up with feeling broken and shattered. My soul is worn out and my spirit is crushed and I'm not sure how much more I can take. I desperately need your closeness. Hold me close. Save me from cancer's blows. No matter what, I trust in your nearness. Come ever closer.

Quenching Our Thirst

Praise be to the God and Father of our Lord Jesus Christ,
the Father of compassion and the God of all comfort,
who comforts us in all our troubles, so that we can
comfort those in any trouble with the comfort
we ourselves receive from God.

2 CORINTHIANS 1:3-4

I'm terrible at hydrating. Most days, I'm oblivious to how thirsty I am until I find myself guzzling a gallon of water as I head to bed. Just as my parched mouth speaks of something to quench it—water—our pain points to something to soothe it—God. He is the God of *all* comfort: the comfort we're given, the comfort we extend to others, the comfort we find in his presence. It's who he is. *God* equals comfort. When we thirst for comfort, God is where we find it. Let's not ignore it.

Lord, let my pain and hurt always lead me to you, the God of all consolation. Thank you not just for being comforting but for being comfort itself. I need it now more than ever, Lord. As you console me in my pain, help me bring solace to others in theirs. Let your comfort overflow in a way I can't contain. For your comfort and compassion, O Lord, I give you thanks.

Jailbreak

He has sent me to bind up the brokenhearted,
to proclaim freedom for the captives and
release from darkness for the prisoners.

ISAIAH 61:1

Whether we're cooped up in bed healing after surgery, missing family gatherings because we're immunosuppressed, or forced to leave our dream job because we can't cope anymore, cancer feels like a dark, damp prison. Trapped, we can allow our mood and outlook to spiral easily into its shadows. Thankfully, Jesus breaks in. He sets us free, bringing light to the blackest nights. Cancer may still be holding us captive, but we've been released from its darkness, set free by our wonderful Father.

Lord, I'm fed up with feeling captive to cancer. I don't want to hurt; I want to heal. I'm done with the shadows of worry and weariness. You came to set me free and release me from this darkness, yet I don't feel free. I don't see your light. Jesus, be my light today. May I know and walk in the freedom I have in you, even if nothing changes. May I see your light in my darkest pain because you have freed me.

His Parting Gift

Peace I leave with you; my peace I give you....
Do not let your hearts be troubled and do not be afraid.

JOHN 14:27

When Jesus died, the disciples appeared to be left alone. Shocked, confused, and seemingly without their leader and guide, they cowered in the upper room. When we feel the same way, let's remember the promise Jesus made to them and us: to leave his peace. It's a peace that stills our hearts, soothes our hurts, and calms our anxieties. Like the disciples, you may feel alone, but you've been given that peace as well. Will you let his peace allay your heartache today?

Lord, you left me your peace, but I often don't feel peaceful. The hurt and pain are just too much. In your presence, shift my suffering into peace. Meet me in my distress. Comfort and calm my aching heart. Remind me how loved I am. I want to go through my day untroubled and unafraid, and in the calm of your presence I can do that. Your parting gift to us was peace, so grant that it may fill me and fuel me today.

Refocus Your Gaze

So we fix our eyes not on what is seen,
but on what is unseen, since what is seen is
temporary, but what is unseen is eternal.

2 CORINTHIANS 4:18

Like a screaming toddler, pain demands our attention and energy. It's hard to ignore a tantruming two-year-old, but the Bible encourages us to turn our eyes away from our pain, no matter how bad it is. I know your hurting is very real, and I'm not dismissing or underestimating it, yet Paul encourages us that it is temporary. Rather than fixating on the pain in front of us, we should, he reminds us, focus on what is unseen ahead: the eternal, the permanent.

Take a moment to refocus your gaze, shifting it from what's here today to the things that will last forever.

Lord, help me take my eyes off the here and now and shift my focus to all you have for me eternally and permanently. I can't do it alone—my pain is too loud and demanding. As I refocus, may I know your eternal love and unfolding grace. Where it feels like I'm falling apart, would you pull me back together?

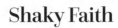

Shaky Faith

"But if you can do anything, take pity on us and help us."
"If you can?" said Jesus. "Everything is possible for one
who believes." Immediately the boy's father exclaimed,
"I do believe; help me overcome my unbelief!"

MARK 9:22-24

It's easy to lose hope when you are hurting. Like the father whose son was regularly thrown into fire or water by a spirit, we wonder whether things will ever change or how we'll get through it. The truth is, no matter how hard things are or how much you're hurting for yourself or someone you love, all things are possible when we believe, no matter how shakily.

Repeat after me: "I believe. Help my unbelief!"

Take pity on me, Lord. My cancer keeps throwing me into the fire and trying to drown me. I've tried everything, and you are my only hope. Strengthen and grow my trust and belief in you—I know you are the great healer. Help me in my doubts and pain. Heal my hurting heart. Mend my broken body. I believe, Lord; help my unbelief.

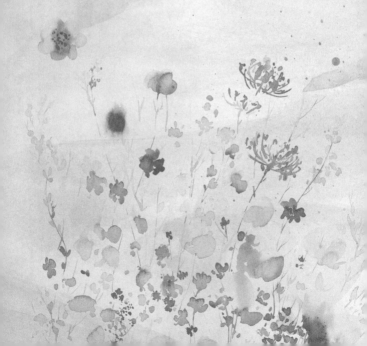

When You're Feeling...

Angry

May your love give me the

strength

to let my anger go.

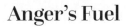

Anger's Fuel

Refrain from anger and turn from wrath;
do not fret—it leads only to evil.

PSALM 37:8

The pain and indignity of treatment, the frustration and resentment at no longer being the women we once were, the time it steals from our precious families—cancer gives us hundreds of reasons to be angry. The emotion can explode suddenly or lurk beneath the surface, smoldering away until we finally erupt. Anger with ourselves, our cancer, and even God is totally understandable. But its energy will always drive us away from God and toward problems. Let's use our anger's fuel to turn toward God rather than away, giving him all our frustrations.

I'm not screaming or raging with anger, Lord, but it simmers, smoldering inside me, constantly steering me away from you. I'm so sorry. As the fire of my anger burns hotter, help me turn to you, confident in your grace and love for me. Strengthen me as I give you my fury. Help me walk in your peace.

Before You Go to Bed

"In your anger do not sin": Do not let the sun go down while you are still angry, and do not give the devil a foothold.

EPHESIANS 4:26-27

Please hear this. Paul isn't saying don't be angry. In fact, anger at injustice is a good thing, and having cancer is most definitely an injustice we must fight. Yet Paul is also clear we are to deal with our anger daily. If we don't, it will overflow into our tomorrows and enable the devil to take advantage of our swirling emotions. Festering anger allowed to simmer overnight only leads to more suffering. So let me ask you this: Do you need to deal with any anger before bedtime tonight?

It's true, Lord, that there are many nights I've pulled up the covers, rolled over, and turned my back on my anger. It's my way of avoiding the issue. I don't want to sin against you or give the enemy a foothold, so help me uncover what's fueling my anger. Give me the courage to let it go and leave it with you. As the sun goes down today, may I sleep in anger-free peace.

Love in Our Anger

Because of the LORD's great love we are not consumed,
for his compassions never fail. They are new
every morning; great is your faithfulness.

LAMENTATIONS 3:22-23

I bet at some point the insensitivity of a doctor, the silence of a friend, or the injustice of your diagnosis has kept you up at night, consumed by hurt and anger. Thankfully, God's love always outweighs our wrath. His compassion means our anger can never totally consume us or shrink us to nothing. He understands, has compassion, and is faithful even in our rage. Our emotions might let us down, but God's love never will. He won't let your anger swallow you completely.

I'm so grateful your unfailing love and compassion arrive fresh each morning. Even as I boil with rage or slowly burn with bitterness, your love and understanding never leave. They always hold me firm. Forgive me for holding fast to my anger and not giving it to you to deal with. As I go into my day, reveal more of your love. Gift me with a greater awareness of your compassion for me. May it be a calming salve to my aching heart.

Soothing Salve

He heals the brokenhearted and binds up their wounds.

PSALM 147:3

Just as a small cut can quickly become infected, inflaming the surrounding skin, our emotional wounds can easily turn angry. We're in pain, our cancer is unfair, and God hasn't fixed it. Unfortunately, as our brokenness and anger lie open and untreated, they slowly morph into fury. Yet even here, with festering wounds, God comes to us and soothes our pain, comforts our sorrow, and binds up our broken hearts.

Today, let's take our angry wounds to the great physician and allow his love to get to work cleaning, bandaging, and healing them.

Lord God, my unresolved hurt and pain have become so infected and raw I'm not sure where the wounds stop and my anger starts. Jesus, I need you. Cleanse the cuts and gashes life and cancer have dealt me. Apply your healing love. Bandage my chipped and cracked heart with your compassion. And grant that I may journey on without the anger that has followed me for far too long.

Undimmable Light

Do everything without grumbling or arguing....
Then you will shine... like stars in the sky.

PHILIPPIANS 2:14-15

Being the nice, well-mannered woman you are, I'm sure you've never had fits of plate-throwing rage or screaming toddler-style tantrums. But if you're like me, your anger seeps out in quick, snarky grumbles or in a long moan on the phone to a friend after a particularly grim procedure. And who hasn't snapped at the smallest thing when they're tired? The trouble is, beneath our grumbling lurks a questioning of God's plans for us, and with each moan, our light, shining into cancer's darkness, slowly dims. So let's take all our moaning and complaints to God and allow his light to shine from us like an undimmable beacon in the night sky.

It's true, Lord, that my anger seeps out when I moan to friends, when I grumble and argue about anything and everything. I'm so sorry. I've let your light within me fade. Every time I want to complain on the phone or pick a fight because I'm mad at the world, show me what I'm doing. Help me stop. May I shine your light and hope to those around me—not darken their days with my moaning.

Absolutely Nothing

For I am convinced that neither death nor life, neither angels nor demons, neither the present nor the future, nor any powers, neither height nor depth, nor anything else in all creation, will be able to separate us from the love of God that is in Christ Jesus our Lord.

ROMANS 8:38-39

If you've ever worried your boiling rage or simmering frustrations will drive a wedge between you and God's love, reread this verse.

God's love for you has absolutely nothing to do with you and everything to do with him. Yes, he is loving, but more than that, he is love itself. It's who he is at his core. He loves you because he loves you, because he is love. Even your anger can't diminish it.

What a relief!

Lord, when I'm angriest, I assume you can't love me—yet you do. Thank you. The depth and strength of your love is unfathomable, but I want to see, taste, and feel more of it. Drown me in your love. Let it fill me to overflowing and wash away my anger. As I grow more convinced of your love each day, may my anger fade away.

Freedom in Forgiveness

*When you stand praying, if you hold
anything against anyone, forgive them, so that
your Father in heaven may forgive you your sins.*

MARK 11:25

When someone says something insensitive or a doctor has the bedside manner of a wet fish, our hurt and anger can grow into full-blown resentment lodged deep inside like a shard of shrapnel.

As Saint Augustine said, clinging to resentment is like drinking poison and waiting for the other person to die, which is why Jesus told us to forgive anyone for anything we hold against them. Not only is unforgiveness unhealthy and unhelpful, but it's also a sin coming between us and God.

Pause as you pray today and forgive anyone you feel resentment toward. As you do, you too will be forgiven.

Lord, I'm sorry for coming to you with all this pent-up resentment still bubbling away inside me. Help me forgive the people who've hurt me. Help me forgive those who have not been there for me, those who have unwittingly said cruel things. I can't do it alone. My resentment has come between us, Lord, but as I forgive others, may I know the closeness and freedom that come from your unconditional love and forgiveness.

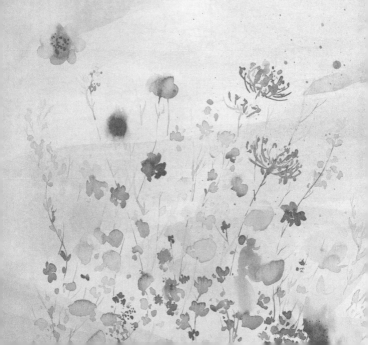

When You're Feeling...

Exhausted

May my tiredness never keep
me from running to you,

Lord.

Watering Our Weariness

*Let my teaching fall like rain and my words
descend like dew, like showers on new grass,
like abundant rain on tender plants.*

DEUTERONOMY 32:2

Have you ever turned your face skyward to let warm summer rain wash away the dust of a long walk? Or maybe you've gulped a cool glass of water to quench a thirst so deep and dry it seemed unshakable. That's how God's Word can work in our lives too. Though our weariness and exhaustion may seem unquenchable, our tender hearts fragile and delicate, his Word refreshes and waters our thirsty, tired souls. In your fatigue, take a moment and sit back, allowing his words to "descend like dew" and refresh every tender part of you today.

Lord, I'm exhausted. My weariness runs so deep and wide it's dried up my hope. It's left me fragile and tenderhearted. Refresh and replenish the driest parts of me with your words and teaching. Let them come like morning dew each day to wake me refreshed. I want to be me again—send your spring showers and revive me. Renew the love and energy I used to know before cancer stripped me bare.

An Invitation to Rest

Because so many people were coming and going that
they did not even have a chance to eat, he said
to them, "Come with me by yourselves
to a quiet place and get some rest."

MARK 6:31

Let's be honest: When we're at our lowest, other human beings—no matter how wonderful and well-meaning—can be exhausting. After a people-filled day, Jesus senses his disciples' exhaustion. He recognizes their need for a break, not to mention something to quieten their growling tummies. In the same way, Jesus always sees and understands how tired, overwhelmed, and yes, even hungry we are, and his response is always the same: to meet us right where we are, offering an invitation to come away with him.

Will you join him?

Lord, I'm so grateful for all the people in my life, and I need them desperately, but it can be exhausting. Thank you for seeing me and understanding. As my mind spins and my body aches, refusing to let me sleep, may I feel your restorative presence. Help me rest in you, Lord. Fill the hungry places within me. More of you, Lord.

Sleep Safe and Sound

In peace I will lie down and sleep,
for you alone, LORD, make me dwell in safety.

PSALM 4:8

How many nights have you lain awake, watching the ceiling fan spin while your mind spirals? Or perhaps your aching body jarred you back into consciousness just as you dozed off. Either way, you're left awake, battling your anxieties and fears. Fear is exhausting. Our cancer, and everything with it, gives us no peace, and we stumble through our days, fear running rampant, feeling anything but safe.

Yet with God, and him alone, we can lie down in safety and peace. Finally—blissfully—sleep comes. Oh, what joy when we've been running on fumes and sleep has seemed so elusive.

Lord, I'm so desperate for sleep. It eludes me. Fitful nights of tossing and turning leave me more exhausted than ever. I'm so over it. Fill me with the peace of knowing I'm safe with you so I can lie down and finally sleep. As I get ready for bed each night, may I know your presence and peace. Calm my racing mind and soothe my aching body, Lord. Remind me how safe I am, and bring sleep to my otherwise sleepless nights.

Renewed Strength

*Those who hope in the L*ORD *will renew their strength.*
They will soar on wings like eagles; they will run and
not grow weary, they will walk and not be faint.

ISAIAH 40:31

Do you worry you *should* be handling things better? Do you feel you *shouldn't* want to hide under the covers, or that you *should definitely* have more get up and go but it's got up and gone? I get it. And thankfully, so does God. Through Isaiah, he reminds us that it doesn't matter who you are or what you're going through—it's okay to feel exhausted. Even healthy young guys and those in their prime get tired and stumble and fall.

Let's not allow our fatigue to rob us of our hope in God, because it's here we'll find our strength renewed. We'll soar, run, walk, and not grow weary. Are you in? I am.

Lord, thank you for understanding how tired I am. Thank you for not giving me a hard time about it. Forgive me for beating myself up when you never do. Lord, I hope in you. Renew my strength. Restore me. May I not grow weary or faint but spread my wings and fly again.

Permanently Replenished

I will refresh the weary and satisfy the faint.

JEREMIAH 31:25

The bone-deep fatigue of cancer isn't just a physical exhaustion. We're emotionally drained, psychologically weary, and often spiritually depleted on top of everything else. As Jeremiah spoke God's words to the people of Israel, he was talking to human beings who, like us, were worn out on every level, who longed to feel alive again. Into this exhaustion, God promised not just momentary refreshment—a glass of lemonade on a summer's day—but full satisfaction and a permanent supply of his living water.

That same promise is for us too. It's for you today, right now.

Lord, I'm bone-tired, on every level: emotionally, physically, and—sad to say—spiritually as well. I need and long for your refreshment and satisfying presence. Fill me up again, Lord. Revive me so I feel alive again, filled with the energy, hope, and expectation of all you have for me. Thank you, Lord, for replenishing me in a way that won't fade or falter but will satisfy my very core, where I need you most.

Our Heavy Lifter

In the same way, the Spirit helps us in our weakness.
We do not know what we ought to pray for, but the Spirit
himself intercedes for us through wordless groans. And he
who searches our hearts knows the mind of the Spirit,
because the Spirit intercedes for God's people
in accordance with the will of God.

ROMANS 8:26-27

If you've ever been exhausted by the thought of praying—what to pray, how to pray, and whether it's even worth it—you're not alone. Thankfully, the Holy Spirit is here to do all the heavy lifting. He translates our wordless groans into prayers and comes alongside us, no matter how weak and weary we are. He searches our hearts before praying for us in line with God's will. We simply need to humbly allow him into our weakness. He'll do the rest.

Lord, I'm sorry my exhaustion has quashed my prayer life. To be honest, I haven't known how, why, or even what to pray. Send your Spirit into my weakness and lack of knowledge. Holy Spirit, as I groan in directionless desperation, transform my mumblings into powerful prayers, and in the presence of God, petition for all I need.

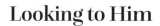

Looking to Him

Look to the LORD and his strength;
seek his face always.

1 CHRONICLES 16:11

I love that you're here, now, reading God's Word and taking time to pray. It's just one way to sit in his presence and seek his face—and it's not always easy to do when we're running on fumes. Yet when we choose to rest in his presence, not only do we see his unending love for us, but we also find his magnificent strength: powerful enough to raise Jesus from the grave and gentle enough to heal the hurting. Strength that is here for us in our weakness.

Whether it's through stillness, worship, Bible study, prayer, or a walk in the woods, can I encourage you to look to him, always?

As you do, you will find that strength.

Lord, I nearly didn't read this devotion today. I'm just too tired. But you've reminded me of your love and strength. Thank you for never hiding your face from me—and for being a God who wants to see mine. As I head into my day, help me look for you at every turn. May I know your strength and power in my weakness and exhaustion.

When You Are...

In a Time of
Waiting

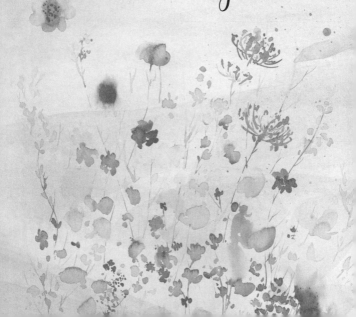

May my waiting be a time
of peace, trust, and
intimacy with you.

Waiting in Hope

The LORD is good to those whose hope is in him,
to the one who seeks him.

LAMENTATIONS 3:25

If your knees are sore and you're all out of words from praying for God to move but he still hasn't shown up, be encouraged. Don't stop or drift away. Keep seeking and hoping, because when you do, whether you see it or not, God is good to you. His goodness might not look like what you're expecting or hoping, but it's always there and rarely more so than when we relentlessly, confidently, passionately, and quietly wait in hope.

Lord, I've had it. I want to give up. Despite my relentless prayers and patient waiting, nothing has changed. You say you're good to me, so help me see and feel your goodness. Show it to me, Lord. My soul longs for you as I seek you in the darkness of this endless waiting. Help me stand firm. Help me continue to hope in you—even when my hope begins to fade and I want to give up. Lead me to where I'll find you, Lord.

Who, Not What

*As for me, I watch in hope for the L̪ᴏʀᴅ,
I wait for God my Savior; my God will hear me.*

MICAH 7:7

The endless soundtrack to my cancer was "Hurry up and wait," and maybe it's yours too. We rush to get a biopsy, then wait endlessly for results. We're raced into surgery before weeks of slow healing. Then there's the waiting and wondering of whether the cancer will return. One minute we're actively fighting, the next we're passively standing by.

But what if your waiting wasn't passive? What if you didn't sit and mark time for your next appointment, result, or call from the doctor but instead watched and waited in hope for the Lord, confident he hears you?

It's not about *what* we're waiting for but *who*.

God, I will wait for you. In this difficult time, help me see my waiting as active forward momentum, not passive inactivity. You are the God of my salvation who hears me, so I won't give up. Meet me in the waiting, Lord. Build hope-filled perseverance in me so I may continue to watch and wait, always in hope.

From What If to What Is

*You will keep in perfect peace those whose minds
are steadfast, because they trust in you.*

ISAIAH 26:3

When we're waiting not just for our kids' soccer practice to be over but for test results that will tell us how many more soccer games we'll be around to watch, our minds wobble and spiral into tailspins of fear-filled what-ifs. Thankfully, it doesn't have to be that way.

Once we set our minds on God, trusting him through the unknowns, we find the peace we long for.

If you're wobbling as you wait, take a moment to refocus away from the what-ifs and toward what is: God. He can be trusted—everything else is a mind game.

Once again, I'm spiraling and battling fear in my waiting, Lord. Forgive me. I've listened to the what-ifs. I've taken my eyes off you and stopped trusting. No wonder I've lost all sense of peace. In the endless waiting, refocus my heart and mind on you. Keep my mind steadfast. As I recommit my heart to who you are and trust you afresh, hold me in your perfect and constant peace.

Stop and Be Still

*Be still before the L<small>ORD</small> and wait patiently for him;
do not fret when people succeed in their ways.*

PSALM 37:7

As you wait, putting life on hold and simply trying to survive, does it seem like everybody else is moving ahead, living their best life? I bet it does! It's easy to get our knickers in a twist and succumb to corrosive, negative emotions: jealousy of others' seemingly fun-filled lives, resentment over everything we're enduring, worry we'll never enjoy life again. Yet God invites us to stop and be still before him, to calm our racing minds and wait patiently for him.

Consider, dear friend, where you are more likely to find peace, in resentful comparison or in stillness before the Lord.

Lord, my mind is pacing, and I'm anything but patient. I see everyone else getting on with their lives while mine has ground to a halt. Calm my racing mind, and forgive my resentful, jealous heart. Help me be still. Teach me to wait patiently for you and you alone. As I give you my fear of being left behind, meet me with your peace and presence. Show me how stillness before you is more precious than speeding after life.

Joy in Joyless Waiting

Be joyful in hope, patient in affliction, faithful in prayer.

ROMANS 12:12

Have you ever met someone whose life is unfathomably hard and painful, yet somehow they're full of joy? How do they do it? Where does this joy come from when their life seems so dark and heavy? Friend, I bet it's from the hope they have in God—a deep, inner confidence in Jesus that bubbles over into hope-filled delight, no matter what happens or what they're waiting for. Today, let me encourage you to have that same confidence in Christ, that same hope. As you do, joy will spring up, and you'll be more patient in pain and more faithful in prayer.

Lord, I can be joyful and rejoice in hope not because of what I'm going through but because of what you've already gone through. When I forget this, remind me. As I struggle to wait, impatient and unfaithful in prayer, help me focus on you. Help me find joy in the hope I have with you and in you alone. Cultivate God-centered confidence in me so my joy, prayers, and patience are fueled by your steadfastness and not reliant on my shifting emotions. May joy overflow in my waiting!

At the Right Times

*The revelation awaits an appointed time....Though it
linger, wait for it; it will certainly come and will not delay.*

HABAKKUK 2:3

If you've ever said, "If I just knew what God was doing," or "Why am I going through this?" you're not alone. The Bible acknowledges that we often won't understand God's purposes in our waiting, and if you're like me, it can drive you bonkers. But it also encourages us to stay the course, certain God will reveal his purposes at the right time. You might be fed up waiting for God's plan, but that doesn't mean it's not coming. Can you wait expectantly? "If it seems slow in coming, wait. It's on its way. It will come right on time."[6]

Your timing is always perfect, Lord. Help me trust you'll reveal your plans when it's time: your time. Forgive my impatience. Teach me to wait with expectancy, confident in your purposes and your schedule. As I wait for you and with you, steady and believing, fill me with peace. Lord, I trust your timing and wait, certain it's on its way.

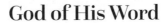

God of His Word

I wait for the LORD, my whole being waits,
and in his word I put my hope.

PSALM 130:5

I just ordered a book online and I had the option for it to arrive in an hour. No waiting required. We live in an instant culture where waiting has become increasingly unnecessary. As a result, we find it more and more uncomfortable. In the kingdom of God, it's different. Waiting is normal, involves our whole being, and is never without hope because God's Word shows us he's a God of his word. He always does what he says he'll do.

Memorize this verse today and cling to it with your entire being, confident his Word never fails.

I know I'm impatient, Lord. I want this cancer to be over and a million other things to happen right this minute. Forgive me. Show me how to wait for you with my entire mind, body, and soul. Strengthen my confidence that you'll show up and do what you've promised so my hope levels increase beyond anything I could manufacture myself. I wait for you, Lord. My whole being waits, and in your Word I put my hope.

When You Are...

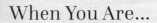
Worrying for
Your Loved Ones

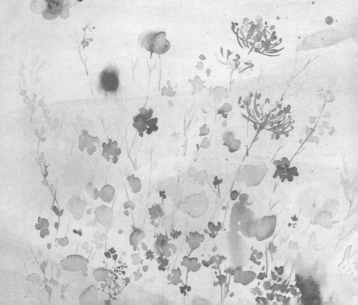

May my worries never eclipse
your *wondrous love.*

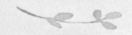

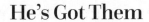

He's Got Them

We love because he first loved us.

1 JOHN 4:19

We worry most for the people we love most. We worry how the kids will react when we lose our hair or how they'll cope with seeing us in the hospital. We worry our husband is short on rest while he's holding down a job (and holding our family together), and we worry for our parents who'd trade places with us in a heartbeat. Our love drives our worry.

So let's remember God loved us first. This love we have for those dearest to us comes from him, and he loves them more passionately than we ever could. He's got them. He always has and always will. No matter what.

Lord, I worry about the people I love most in this world, about the million ways my cancer will affect them. Your unending love that loved me first fuels this worry, so help me remember its depth and breadth—for me and for them. Help me entrust my precious people into your loving care, and grant that we may all find the peace and strength we need in you.

Parent, Protector, Provider

A father to the fatherless, a defender of widows, is God
in his holy dwelling. God sets the lonely in families.

PSALM 68:5-6

Now that you have cancer, do you feel like you're failing the people you love most? It's understandable. The bedtime stories, wedding showers, girls' nights out, graduations, and family dinners we miss leave a gaping hole. And what if it becomes permanent?

It's hard for sure, but always remember God commits to watch over our loved ones. He steps in as parent, protector, and provider, promising to place the lonely within families of love. He pledges to fill that void emotionally, spiritually, and physically. Who better to do the job than the creator of the universe!

Lord God, it's as if I've fallen off the planet. I'm missing so much and feel so absent and removed from the people I love. Thank you for being there for them. Thank you for promising your presence both now and if and when this cancer takes everything from them. In my worry, remind me of all you are and all you will do to fill this void, so I can rest and recuperate in peace. Fill the gaps I'm leaving, Lord.

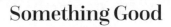

Something Good

*We know that in all things God works
for the good of those who love him.*

ROMANS 8:28

Unfortunately, God never promised us a trouble-free life, one without pain, heartache, loneliness, or hurt. He does, however, promise to work for our good in the midst of it all, including cancer. I know quoting this verse can sound trite—like an empty Christian platitude—but at its core is God's love for you and your nearest and dearest.

No matter what cancer throws at you, you can be sure that "every detail in our lives of love for God is worked into something good."[7] Today, will you trust God to do that for everyone you love?

Lord, I am clinging to your promise to use for good anything and everything cancer throws at us. Right now, I can't see how you'll do that or what good can come of it, but I'm deciding to walk into today believing it's true. May this suffering not be for nothing.[8] Bring beauty and goodness from the pain and heartache cancer has given my precious people. Help them see it and know it, today and always.

The Safest Hands

My Father, who has given them to me, is greater than all;
no one can snatch them out of my Father's hand.

JOHN 10:29

I bet you're a brilliant mom. You held your kids close when they grazed a knee, fell out with friends, or headed off to college. As moms, we can't imagine a safer place for them than secure in our arms. I don't want to burst your bubble, but God's hands are greater still! They're the safest place our kids can be, no matter what. Before you pray, I invite you to take a moment to close your eyes and visualize placing your precious children into his hands, confident that no one will snatch them away.

Lord, forgive me for forgetting your hands are safer and more secure than mine, for thinking I'm all my children need to be okay. Your hands are the best place they can ever be. Thank you for never letting them go. Thank you for loving them even more than I do. Today I place them in your hands, choosing your arms over mine for them, entrusting them to you. Watch over and protect them. Give them all they need.

Getting Out of the Way

*Jesus said, "Let the little children come to me,
and do not hinder them, for the kingdom of
heaven belongs to such as these."*

MATTHEW 19:14

As moms we long for our kids to run to Jesus unhindered, yet we're often the very obstacle getting in their way. In our worry we hold them too close or tell them they're strong and can cope alone. I'm not saying don't hold your kids or tell them they'll be okay. But we become the barrier when we choose to do that over and above encouraging them to go to Jesus.

Remember, the kingdom of heaven belongs to them, so let's not let our worries get in their way.

Father, I never thought my intense love for my kids might stop them from coming to you, but I guess it could. Forgive me. I never intended to get in their way. Thank you for the gift of your kingdom. May my kids come to you freely and eagerly, especially when they're worried or upset. Increase my confidence in your love for them and grant that my love may always steer them toward you.

Help When We're Hiding

*I lift up my eyes to the mountains—where does
my help come from? My help comes from the
L<small>ORD</small>, the Maker of heaven and earth.*

PSALM 121:1-2

Cancer is a roller coaster of emotions. One minute we're strong, motivated, and ready to tackle it head-on, but the next—driven by worry about those we love—we're weak, helpless, hopeless, and ready to hide under the duvet.

From our hiding places, let's lift our eyes to the mountains, remembering who God is: the creator of everything, the place we find help when we're most helpless. Whether you're surrounded by skyscrapers, dry desert, or flat prairies, can you lift your mind's eye to the mountains, confident help is on the way?

I hate feeling helpless, God. Cancer has stolen the capable, strong woman I was, and it infuriates me. Yet you are here and you love me. Help me take my gaze off myself and rest it on you. As I look to the mountains, may I be reassured of your help and provision, not just for me but for everyone I love so dearly. Be my help. Be their help. Be our everything.

God's Protection

*Have you not put a hedge around him
and his household and everything he has?*

JOB 1:10

The protection a hedge offers sounds pretty puny to me (wouldn't you rather have a concrete bunker?), but in biblical times hedges were put around flocks at night to protect them from wild predators and thieves. God set a hedge of protection around Job and his family, and he continues to do the same for us today. As we think about our loved ones, let's pray for a towering, impenetrable hedge—as strong as reinforced steel—around them.

Lord, you are our protection. Set a mighty hedge around my most precious people and protect them from everything coming against them. As night closes in, may they rest in the knowledge they are safe with you, confident you are there, will never leave, and are their biggest defender. As we journey through these difficult days, may we know and see your love and protection each and every moment.

When You Are...

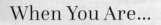

Uncertain About the Future

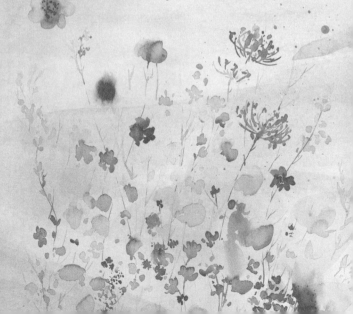

Stumbling into uncertainty,
may I know the certainty of your
loving presence.

Stepping Ahead

In their hearts humans plan their course,
but the LORD establishes their steps.

PROVERBS 16:9

You're a capable, make-it-happen woman. You have calendars, schedules, plans, and action lists to help you stay focused and get stuff done. Unfortunately, as cancer takes over and plans fall apart, a disconcerting out-of-control feeling, a sense of being adrift, can become constant.

It's not that we shouldn't make plans. It's just unwise to do so without seeking God first. He alone establishes our steps, and his ways are always better than ours. In our nervousness about what's around the corner, let's not jump ahead of God.

How can you let him choose your steps today?

All my wonderful plans for the days, weeks, months, and even years ahead have been thrown in the air by this diagnosis. I feel so untethered, God. I want to make plans. I have things to look forward to, things to put in place for my family, but I know I can easily jump ahead of you. Lord, don't let me do that. Show me your course and establish my steps so I might walk into the future secure with you.

Standing Firm in Love

Be on your guard; stand firm in the faith;
be courageous; be strong. Do everything in love.

1 CORINTHIANS 16:13-14

As a planner and self-appointed make-it-happen captain, I felt my fuse snap the moment cancer pulled the rug out from under my well-ordered, planned-out life. Let's just say I wasn't always my most gracious, loving, faith-filled self. Yet amid the uncertainty, *who* we are as a person is just as important as *what* we do.

Now more than ever, when we'd probably be forgiven for taking our fear and frustrations out on others, we need to be on our guard, stand firm, be strong, and do everything in love. Thankfully, the more we stand firm in God, the easier we find it.

How can you stand on his love today? What do you need to do in love?

Lord, I know I've been taking my fear and frustrations out on others. I'm sorry. As the ground beneath me shakes and I try to stand firm, hold me fast. Help me choose courage and strength over fear. Grant that I may "love without stopping" today.[9]

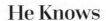

He Knows

"I know the plans I have for you," declares the Lord,
*"plans to prosper you and not to harm you,
plans to give you hope and a future."*

JEREMIAH 29:11

D o you feel captive to cancer, robbed of the future
you'd planned and imagined? I did. This familiar
verse can seem like an empty platitude, but it was spo-
ken to the people of Israel during their captivity in Bab-
ylon. Like you, they felt cheated out of the future God
had promised.

The truth is, we can never know what the future
holds, so it's vital to remember that God knows. There
is never a time when he doesn't have plans for you. God
says, "I have it all planned out—plans to take care of you,
not abandon you, plans to give you the future you hope
for."[10] What amazing reassurance for facing the uncertain days ahead.

*Lord, I hate not knowing what's before me, but I'm re-
assured and grateful you do. Build my trust and hope
in this truth. May I live in this place of uncertainty with
peaceful assurance, certain your plans flow from your
love and are good, even when life isn't. In my captivity,
show me your goodness.*

Stop Figuring It Out

Trust in the Lord with all your heart and lean not on your own understanding; in all your ways submit to him, and he will make your paths straight.

PROVERBS 3:5-6

BC (before cancer) it was easy to trust our heads and hearts as we went along, charting our own course. Then cancer stormed in, throwing everything in the air and leaving us stumbling through the darkness of our new lives.

Yes, we may feel lost, on a path too dark and windy to navigate, but the Lord promises to guide us. Ironically, we find our way when we stop trying to figure it out. Once we stop relying on what we think we know and give in to God, who does know, he makes the way forward clear. He keeps us on track.

Lord, I tend to trust myself more than you—to chart my path and figure out the future alone. I'm sorry. As I head into the unknown, may I rely on you with all my heart. Lead me in every decision. Keep me on track today and always. Help me submit to you and grow my trust in you.

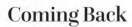

Coming Back

*Remain in me, as I also remain in you. No branch
can bear fruit by itself; it must remain in the vine.
Neither can you bear fruit unless you remain in me.*

JOHN 15:4

We all want our lives to be fruitful, to have a clear sense of purpose and meaning, and, despite appearances, cancer doesn't rob us of this gift. It might just look different now. Cancer can't stop us bearing fruit. Only uncoupling ourselves from Jesus can do that.

Maybe, in the unpredictability and uncertainty of life since your diagnosis, you've drifted away. If so, can I invite you to come back to that place of abiding in him? It's at home with Jesus that we find clarity.

Lord, thank you for remaining in me even when, in my uncertainty and fear of the future, I drift away from you. As I come back to you today, make your home in me anew. Grow fruit within me and around me that gives you all the glory. Help me see the fresh, tender fruit I need to tend. And if I do start to drift away again, Lord, hold me tighter still.

Seeing in the Dark

Your word is a lamp for my feet, a light on my path.

PSALM 119:105

C ancer leaves us fumbling in the dark, scrabbling in the inky blackness of our disease, unsure where to step next.

Down the ages, ordinary Christians like us have discovered that no matter how black the days may be, God's Word helps us see in the dark. The future may be uncertain, but his Word throws light onto the murky road ahead.

Sometimes I wish God's lamp was bigger or stronger, one that lit my path off into the distance and not just around my feet. But experience has taught me his beam is always enough to see where to step next.

I'm lost in total darkness here, Lord, and I need you to illuminate my path. Forgive me for trying to light the way with other things. They'll never love me like you do or shine as brightly as your Word. As I read your Word today, would you speak, guiding me forward? I'm listening and will follow. As everything falls apart and I fumble, lost in the gloom, may your Word always hold me together, lighting my way.

Rubies in the Rubble

Do not worry about tomorrow, for tomorrow will worry about itself. Each day has enough trouble of its own.

MATTHEW 6:34

In your worrying about tomorrow, are you perhaps in danger of missing everything today has to offer? Yes, today might be a horrid day, but there's still goodness buried here—if we look. When we spend our time in a tizzy about what may or may not happen tomorrow, we miss today's rubies buried in the rubble of our cancer-shaken life. After all, God will help us handle whatever tomorrow holds, so let's not let it rob us of our todays. How can you be more present today, right here, right now?

Lord, forgive me for fixating on tomorrow when today, in all its goodness, is right in front of me. Help me be present and enjoy what you're doing each moment. Help me notice the beauty buried in the rubble of my life and see the joy in front of me. I trust I'll be able to cope with whatever comes tomorrow because you are with me. May I live today in the peace that knowledge brings.

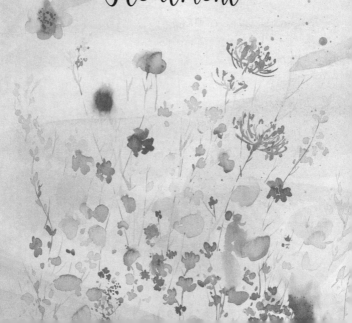

When You Are...

Going Through
Treatment

As treatment weakens

my ailing body,

strengthen me

with your eternal love.

He'll See You Through

The LORD replied, "My Presence
will go with you, and I will give you rest."

EXODUS 33:14

Starting months of treatment is like setting off into an unforgiving desert of scorching days, freezing nights, and battles against unknown enemies. As Moses and the Israelites set off through their wilderness, God gave them his ultimate comfort—the promise of his presence in the journey ahead—and he gives it to you too. In your journey through treatment, God's constant, unshifting presence through Jesus is with you, and with that presence comes the rest you so desperately need. The next time you walk into chemo or have surgery, take a minute to remember God is there and will see you through.

Lord God, looking ahead to my treatment, I'm grateful for your promise to go with me and give me rest. In my exhaustion and worry, I need your presence desperately. As they pump me full of chemo, infuse me with your peace. As I'm wheeled into surgery, may I know your nearness. And as I recuperate, rebuilding my strength day by day, would you help me rest and restore my soul? Lord, I trust you'll see me through.

Your Lifeguard and Firefighter

When you pass through the waters, I will be with you;
and when you pass through the rivers, they will not sweep
over you. When you walk through the fire, you will not
be burned; the flames will not set you ablaze.

ISAIAH 43:2

Does it feel like you've stepped into a raging river and a roaring furnace at the same time? Treatment makes us feel as if we're simultaneously drowning and burning up, constantly in need of both a firefighter and a lifeguard. Thankfully, in Jesus, we have just that. God promises to be our Savior—both firefighter and lifeguard—who will never leave us to be swept away by torrents or consumed by flames. As you pass through the fiery waters of treatment, he'll get you through.

There are days, Lord, when it all feels too much. The nausea and pain consume me, and any energy, hope, or joy I had is swept away. I'm running on fumes. But you are my Savior. I trust you'll never leave me or let the fires and waters of treatment totally overwhelm me. Hold me above the river; protect me from the flames. Get me through, Lord. I need you today.

Extravagant Love, Explosive Power

I pray that out of his glorious riches he may strengthen you
with power through his Spirit in your inner being, so that
Christ may dwell in your hearts through faith.

EPHESIANS 3:16-17

Treatment doesn't just beat up our bodies—it sucker punches our deepest places. In fact, fighting cancer physically makes it easy to forget our innermost beings—our tender, emotional, and spiritual places—need just as much strengthening and healing as our outer bodies.

As you go through treatment, why not pray along with Paul and ask God to flood those tender parts of you? Not only will you be able to take hold of the "extravagant dimensions of Christ's love" (MSG), but you can also anticipate the unlimited strength, the "divine might and explosive power" (TPT) you have through his Spirit.

Everything within me is tired, hurting, anxious, and confused, Lord. The more my body takes a pounding, the more my tenderest places take a battering—and the more my mind, will, and emotions weaken. Help me see the unlimited heavenly blessings I have in you. Show me the enormity of your love, and refuel and refill me from the inside out. I need your strength and resolve. I can't battle on without them.

Honesty

My life is consumed by anguish and my years
by groaning; my strength fails because of
my affliction, and my bones grow weak.

PSALM 31:10

D o you worry God isn't interested in your troubles, perhaps assuming he's got more important things to worry about (like global warming), he's mad about the mess you've made of your life, or he's simply written you off as not spiritual enough to make his action list? Thankfully, that's all rubbish! God loves you and wants to hear your struggles, just as they are, in all their pain and ugliness. Like the psalmist, why not pour out your frustration and pain to God? I promise you he can take it and it won't make him love you any less.

I'm sorry I haven't told you how hurt, angry, confused, and worried I am. Forgive me for seeing you as a fickle and irate God, as an unloving Father who doesn't care about his children. Thank you for always listening and never rejecting me. Lord, I'm exhausted. I've cried myself to sleep more times than I can count, and I don't remember when I last felt strong and alive. I'm over it. Help me, Lord. Strengthen me.

Your Home

Whoever dwells in the shelter of the Most High
will rest in the shadow of the Almighty.

PSALM 91:1

During treatment, our doctor's office and chemo ward quickly become our second homes, but we hope they are just short-term rentals and not long-term residences. Unfortunately, during our time there, we're permanently exhausted and anxious.

What if we could change that?

What if, no matter what we faced or where we sat, God's presence was our home? Well, my friend, it can be. Just because you're "dwelling" in the hospital after surgery, or lying in bed after another round of chemo, doesn't mean you can't sit in his sheltering presence. And when you do, you'll always find rest.

Today, how can you still yourself before him and soak up his peace?

Lord, even while I sit in the chemo chair or lie on a scanner, my heart and soul live and rest in your sheltering presence. As I curl into bed, help me rest in your shadow and find the peace and strength I long for. Lord, may I focus less on the building, and the bed I'm in, and more on whose presence I sit in. Fill me with your rest, Lord.

The Gift of Weakness

He gives strength to the weary
and increases the power of the weak.

ISAIAH 40:29

I hate feeling weak, either physically or emotionally. I assume I shouldn't be so pathetic and wonder why I can't just pull myself together and get on with life. Then I remember: It's only in this place of weakness that God can strengthen us.

When there isn't a chink in our armor and we've got it all figured out, it's easy to assume we don't need God, so we forge ahead alone, missing out on his power. Our fragility is our greatest gift. Our lack of power enables God to energize us with his.

Surely that's better than anything we can do ourselves?

As you endure the weakness and frailty of treatment, remember God promises not just to strengthen you but to increase your power. How wonderful—and how great is our God!

Lord Jesus, I hate feeling weak. I'm ashamed of my tissue-thin strength to hold myself together on my own, but so thankful it's here you can do what you do best. Jesus, pour out your strength and power on me today. In my tiredness and stumbling, restore my energy. Refuel my aching body.

God's Sustaining Gift

*He will wipe every tear from their eyes. There will be
no more death or mourning or crying or pain,
for the old order of things has passed away.*

REVELATION 21:4

The Bible doesn't tell us much about heaven, but what we know for sure is that there'll be no suffering—no crying or death, no heartache, pain, or loss. Doesn't that sound wonderful?

God could have told us so much more, but this is the one thing we know for certain. I often wonder why. I've come to believe this picture of a pain-free heaven awaiting us —hopefully years in the future—is a gift to sustain us in today's suffering.

No matter what, you can be sure of two things: God is with you now, and one day, when a whole new order is here, there'll be no pain or suffering. Amen!

Lord, this sustaining image of heaven with you, where we're free of pain and hurt, is wonderful. I want my suffering to be over now, but until it is, may this image strengthen and sustain me. When the tears flow steadily and the pain penetrates deeply, fill my heart with your heavenly hope.

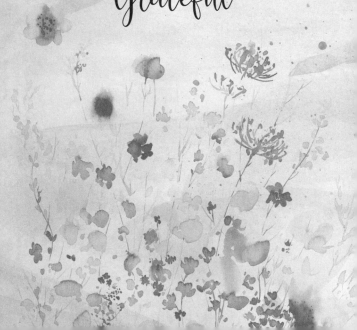

When You Are...

Relieved and
Grateful

No storm can diminish your
goodness, so may I
give thanks
come rain or shine.

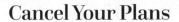

Cancel Your Plans

The LORD has done it this very day;
let us rejoice today and be glad.

PSALM 118:24

Yes, we're meant to rejoice in the good news of the gospel—whether our days are bursting with sunshine and roses or stink worse than a teenager's PE kit. But honestly, some moments are easier to celebrate than others. Cancer isn't exactly known for its abundance of encouraging times, so when we hit a bright spot, let's revel in it.

Today is one of those days. Why? Because you know the blessing of the Lord and what he's done. So cancel your plans, put everything aside, and rejoice and be glad in it.

Today is a good day. I can hardly believe it. I'm happy, grateful, and relieved for the first time in ages, so I rejoice and give you praise. After enduring days of worry and hurting, I can see this moment for what it is: a bright spot shining brilliantly among the shadows. So help me celebrate, Lord—not just in today's news (although it is pretty wonderful) but in the enduring good news of the gospel and what you've done for me. Let's celebrate!

Our Father of Lights

*Every good and perfect gift is from above,
coming down from the Father of the heavenly lights,
who does not change like shifting shadows.*

JAMES 1:17

Whether your scan shows your tumor has shrunk, it's your final day of treatment, or your kid got into their top college choice, good news is a welcome ray of sunshine in the dark, cloudy days of cancer. These blessings today, illuminating your path and lightening your load, come from the Father of lights himself. His light never dims, flickers, or goes out. He never changes.

As you celebrate today's news and feel the tingle of hope it brings, remember there are more good and perfect gifts to come, because that is who he is!

Lord God, as I walk through the shifting shadows of my cancer journey, I'm grateful for your gifts lighting my way. May I never forget how unchanging you are. And no matter how dark things get, may you always be the beacon toward which I walk: my guiding light. Thank you for today's gift, and in anticipation, thank you for all your gifts to come.

Our Whole Selves

In view of God's mercy...offer your bodies
as a living sacrifice, holy and pleasing to God—
this is your true and proper worship.

ROMANS 12:1

How does the saying go? "God is good all the time. All the time God is good." It's true but easy to forget when you're in the middle of cancer. So when our load is lighter and life is easier, let's be sure to respond appropriately to God's grace. Here Paul tells us we do that by offering our whole selves to him afresh. And remember, no matter how you choose to give yourself to God today, he'll love it.

Lord, you're so kind, generous, and merciful. I deserve nothing from you, yet you gave everything for me. Today I'm placing before you, as an offering, my everyday, ordinary life—my sleeping, eating, going-to-work, and walking-around life, as well as my cancer-journey life. Embracing what you've done for me is the best thing I can do for you, and it's something that, with your help, I can accomplish.[11] Accept my gift of thanks, today and always.

Give It Away

Give, and it will be given to you.

LUKE 6:38

Since you're reading a devotion about feeling relief and gratitude, I'm assuming you've had some good news. I'm delighted and celebrating at my desk.

As you sink into the relief and enjoy a smile creasing the corners of your eyes, let me ask you this: How can you share this goodness? How can you give it away?

Who can you encourage? Is there someone you can text or make a meal for? Can you pray for others who might not have received good news as you have?

Remember, it's in the giving that we receive, and what we receive is far more than we can ever give.

Lord, I'm sitting in relief, and for once, I'm not drowning in worry. Thank you. You are the God we can't outgive, so show me how to give this goodness to others. Lead me to those who need practical help or an encouraging word. I lift to you everyone who's feeling the weight of worry that hasn't been lifted by good news. Where they're running on empty, fill and strengthen them. Heal them and give them hope when it feels hopeless.

A Habit of Gratitude

Give thanks in all circumstances;
for this is God's will for you in Christ Jesus.

1 THESSALONIANS 5:18

Whether they're good, bad, or ugly, our circumstances mustn't dictate our levels of gratitude. If today is a good day, let's be cheerful and thank God. And if tomorrow's a painful mess, let's be grateful then too, because it's our calling—to give thanks always, no matter what.

God wants us to practice gratitude through thick and thin because it always blesses us. When we give thanks, we see our circumstances differently, so let's start to make gratitude a habit today, when things are good. It will make giving thanks in harder times easier.

Today I feel lighter, Lord, and I thank you. Your will for me is good, pleasing, and perfect (Romans 12:2) no matter what, so I pledge to give thanks—not just today but always. As I do, change my heart to see things as you see them, shifting my outlook from the shadows around me to your light above me. Today is good, but when it's not, help me see both the rubies and the rubble of my life and give thanks for it all.

Oil and Water

A time to weep and a time to laugh,
a time to mourn and a time to dance.

ECCLESIASTES 3:4

I used to think emotions were like oil and water, with differing feelings unable to mix. Cancer taught me otherwise. Panic and peace, hope and fear, mourning and dancing, crying and laughing—they can all coexist and be fully present together.

In the midst of cancer, if we waited to celebrate until we're totally happy—without an ounce of worry or pain—we'd never pop the poppers or raise a glass.

So please don't let your lingering grief or nagging fear stop you from laughing, cheering, and boogying. As the T-shirts say, "Life is good." Let's relax and party.

I don't understand how it works, Lord, but I'm a jumble of contradictory emotions. In there somewhere is relief and gratitude, so no matter what else I feel, I praise you. In the midst of my crying, help me giggle like a child. As I grieve my many losses, show me how to dance in your goodness. With you, there's a right time for it all, and today I'm grateful that time is now.

When You Are...

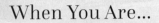
Facing a Setback

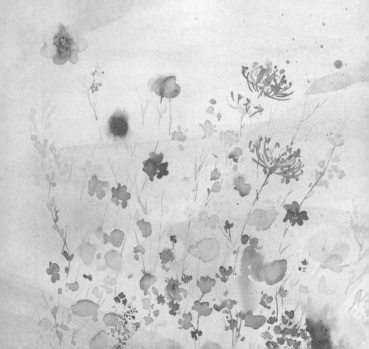

May I continuously

move forward

with you.

Who and What We Trust

When I am afraid, I put my trust in you. In God,
whose word I praise—in God I trust and am not afraid.

PSALM 56:3-4

I doubt anyone has journeyed through cancer seamlessly, progressing from diagnosis to remission, or even cure, without a hiccup or setback. Yet don't we long for and maybe even secretly expect it? So much so that with the arrival of setbacks—complications from surgery or the departure of a loved and trusted doctor—we spiral backward. All forward momentum gone, we're left facing a chasm of uncertainty.

This is the time to focus on what we do know, not what we don't. On who and what we can trust—God and his Word. The Word of God never sets us back! When we return to him, trusting and praising his promises, we have nothing to fear.

Lord, everything seemed fine, until this. It feels like I've taken one step forward and five back. In my turmoil, I return to you and your Word. Strengthen my faith in you and your promises. As I trust you and praise your promises, may my fear fade away.

Somehow, Someday

I will repay you for the years the locusts have eaten.

JOEL 2:25

Battling cancer is hard enough, but the relentless skirmishes and setbacks that go with it are enough to make the strongest woman want to give up. Frightening test results, mounting medical bills, and lengthy complications darken our days like clouds of swarming locusts, consuming our energy, finances, health, and hope. In their midst you may feel unseen and forgotten. But you're not. God not only sees us cowering from the onslaught but promises to restore everything that's been devoured. He knows the intimate details of your loss. You can trust he'll make up for it. Somehow. Some day.

Do you really see what cancer has stolen from me, Lord? Here in the darkness of one setback after another, it doesn't always feel like it. So today I'm going to choose to believe you. I'm going to choose to live in the confidence of your promise. Even if I can't imagine how you'll repay me—and no matter whether it's this side of heaven or not—may I stand taller, stronger, and more hope-filled in the face of today's news. Lord, fuel me with faith.

Everlasting Hope

*Return to your fortress, you prisoners of hope; even now
I announce that I will restore twice as much to you.*

ZECHARIAH 9:12

Do you feel knocked back to the place you thought you'd broken free from? Maybe you're back in the chemo chair after getting the all clear or simply back in bed after thinking your energy had returned. Setbacks make us feel trapped, prisoners to our disease.

Remember, though, you might *feel* like a prisoner of cancer, captive to despair, but in reality you're a prisoner of hope, and this everlasting hope is independent of how your cancer journey is going. Listen to the cry of the prophet Zechariah and come back to your fortress: the fortress of hope. It is yours and yours forever.

Lord, your hope gets knocked out of me when I get knocked back. It's worrying how easily it vanishes and how far I drift from the safety of your fortress. Today I come back. Restore the security and peace of the confidence I have in you. In my returning, may hope rise up. May I see your restoration.

Fill Me Afresh

The Spirit God gave us does not make us timid,
but gives us power, love and self-discipline.

2 TIMOTHY 1:7

Wouldn't it be great if life, even in its toughest parts, unfolded in the orderly, linear way we planned? Unfortunately, that's rarely the case. Just as Timothy did, we face setbacks, detours, dead ends, and difficulties, and Paul reminds us, in the same way he did Timothy, to never forget we have God's Spirit within us, a ready source of power, love, and self-discipline. We might feel afraid or even cowardly in the face of cancer's constant pounding, but God's Spirit will calm and strengthen us.

Take a moment to invite God to fill you with his Spirit afresh today.

To be honest, Lord, these constant disappointments spiral me into fear. In my struggles, fill me with your Spirit. Equip me to face cancer from within, overflowing with your power, love, and self-discipline, not drowning in weakness, fear, and self-indulgence. Your Spirit always leads to hope and calm. Help me walk tall in those gifts today.

Return to Center

Submit yourselves, then, to God.
Resist the devil, and he will flee from you.

JAMES 4:7

If you've ever watched a tennis match, you'll have seen that no matter where an opponent's shot took them, the players always return to the center of the court. Just like a tennis pro, when setbacks send us way out of bounds, we must focus first on coming back to our center, God, and submitting to him. The devil won't miss a chance to cause trouble and send us running, but when we resist him, he *will* flee!

How has the enemy sent you sprinting? How can you make a stand against his works and submit yourself to God today? When you're back at the center of the court with God, you'll be able to handle anything.

Lord, forgive me for letting the enemy lure me away from you. As I return, help me give you full access to my life. I say yes to you and no to the devil. I want to be ready for the next time the enemy attacks, so strengthen and equip me, Lord.

Pressing On

One thing I do: Forgetting what is behind and
straining toward what is ahead, I press on toward
the goal to win the prize for which God has
called me heavenward in Christ Jesus.

PHILIPPIANS 3:13-14

Have you've ever groaned, "Ugh, not again," or "I thought I was doing so much better," or even "Remember what happened last time we tried that?" If you have, then you know how cancer's setbacks can dictate how we move forward.

Despite having more stumbling blocks than you and I have had hot dinners, Paul managed to leave them behind and press on toward all God had for him. How? He knew Jesus intimately, was confident of God's love and grace, and let nothing else distract him. Not even the past.

Whether this is your first or five hundredth setback, can you keep your eyes on the prize, on Jesus, the one God calls you to seek?

Lord, I fixate on the knocks and disappointments, not on you. Forgive me. Help me forget them and fix my eyes, heart, and hope on what's ahead—you and your prize. You reached out to me, so now I reach for you.

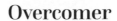

Overcomer

In this world you will have trouble.
But take heart! I have overcome the world.

JOHN 16:33

Jesus is clear: Our lives won't be perfect and pain-free. Yet we're still surprised when they're not. Perhaps subconsciously we believe we're invincible or think our "good behavior" gives us a get-out-of-suffering-free card. Regardless, it means we quickly lose heart when things don't turn out as we'd hoped.

So let's remind ourselves of Jesus's triumph and how he conquered the world. Yes, things are going to be hard, but thanks to Christ, we can have hope, be encouraged, and take heart. Remember, my friend, in him you too are an overcomer.

Lord, I'm sorry I get so discouraged when things don't go as planned, when scans or tests set me back—again. You never said life would be trouble free, and yet, somehow, I always expect it to be. Forgive me. Encourage my tired and struggling heart today, Lord. Remind me of how you overcame the world and how, with you, I might do the same. With you, I can face anything. With you, I can take heart.

When You're Wrestling
with Faith...

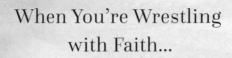

And Questioning God

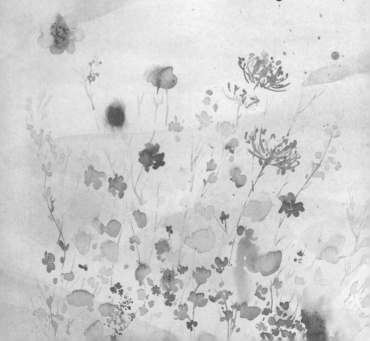

May my questioning
always draw me
closer to you.

Cry Out with Confidence

Why, Lord, do you stand far off?
Why do you hide yourself in times of trouble?

PSALM 10:1

Have you've ever screamed, *God, where are you when I need you? Are you avoiding me?* If so, you're not alone. A quick skim through some Psalms assures us we're not the first—and probably won't be the last—to question God. Yet the psalmists were confident of a couple things we easily forget: It's okay to question God, and even if God seems far off or hiding, he's not.

Today, if you find yourself questioning whether God has vanished or is avoiding you, take your lead from the psalmist and cry out to your Creator with confidence. He welcomes your honesty and hasn't turned his back on you.

It feels like you've abandoned me, Lord. Like you're standing far off, turning your back, and hiding your face. Are you? I need you now more than ever. I can't do this alone. Strengthen my confidence in your presence. Continually reassure me that you're not angered by my cries, that you won't turn away from me. Fill me with your peace today, Lord, no matter what.

Unafraid to Ask

*If any of you lacks wisdom, you should ask God,
who gives generously to all without finding
fault, and it will be given to you.*

JAMES 1:5

A cancer diagnosis can leave the wisest, most confident woman reeling and confused—and let's not pretend chemo brain and cancer fog aren't real! They'll dampen our sharp, quick-thinking minds faster than we can say "What day is it?" leaving us exhausted and questioning everything and everyone, especially God.

We long for clarity in our faith, but there are days we lack the capacity to choose what socks to wear, let alone figure out theological conundrums. Thankfully, when we ask God for guidance and insight, he doesn't see our lack of wisdom as a fault. No, he loves to help and gives generously. So let's not be afraid to ask.

*I can't seem to form a clear thought or make a wise
decision, and I'm paralyzed by indecision and doubt.
Especially about you, Lord. I need your help and wisdom.
Show me the way forward, guiding and leading me
through difficult decisions and my questioning faith.*

The Ultimate Google

*Call to me and I will answer you and tell you
great and unsearchable things you do not know.*

JEREMIAH 33:3

Google has the answer to pretty much everything, but there's much about God that's ungoogleable: unsearchable, even in the depths of the world's collective knowledge. At times that's comforting, at others, deeply frustrating. When much of our cancer journey is unknown, we long for both our medical and faith questions to be answered, and it's mind-blowing to think the God who made the earth and all things in it invites us to ask him. "I'll tell you marvelous and wondrous things that you could never figure out on your own."[12] Wow!

Your Creator is saying, "I'm the ultimate Google. Use me!" Let's take our questions about God to him, not Google.

There is so much I long to know for certain, God. Cancer has shaken my world and faith, and I'm searching for answers. I'm desperate to find solid ground beneath my feet. Show me what I don't know. Tell me things I can't search for alone, and reveal the wonderful mysteries I could never figure out without you. May my questioning draw me closer to you and your answers always fuel my faith.

Filled to Overflowing

I pray that you, being rooted and established in love, may have power... to know this love that surpasses knowledge—that you may be filled to the measure of all the fullness of God.

EPHESIANS 3:17-19

It can feel like God slipped out the back door the moment cancer barged through the front, and in the resulting pain and struggle, it's easy to assume he's gone for good. Thankfully, no matter how it seems, we've been promised otherwise. God's love for us is so huge it goes beyond any human knowledge or understanding. It's an extravagant love that doesn't leave the moment things get dicey but instead fills us to overflowing with all of who he is.

Can you see how, in the midst of your cancer, God is showing you the depths of that love?

Before I was diagnosed, I didn't seem to question your love or presence, Lord, but now I do, more and more. I'm sorry. Root me in your love again so that I'm sure of you beside me and within me. Astonish me with the depth and breadth of your love that my life may be full to overflowing with the extraordinary, expansive extravagance of it.

Questioning Our Questions

Dear friends, do not believe every spirit,
but test the spirits to see whether they are from God.

1 JOHN 4:1

My husband, Al, always says there are four sound-tracks or voices we listen to as we go through life: our own thoughts, the messages of the world, the enemy's lies, and the voice of God. Yes, cancer leaves us with questions and doubts, with thoughts about God, the future, and more, but let's make sure we know where they're coming from.

I'm not saying questioning God is bad, but we must make sure we're not believing the rubbish being thrown at us by the world, the enemy, or even our own minds. Next time you're questioning God, ask yourself one thing: Is this consistent with the Bible and with love? If not, it's probably not God. Friend, let's test the questioning spirits!

I have a million thoughts, questions, worries, doubts, and concerns every moment of every day, Lord, and I need your help to see what is from you. Deafen my ears to anything except your voice. Highlight what is from you, and silence the lies and wonderings the enemy whispers cunningly to me. Grant that my ears may always be tuned to your heartbeat.

Our God of Order

God is not a God of disorder but of peace.

1 CORINTHIANS 14:33

Cancer shakes our well-ordered lives into a chaotic mess of unpredictable moving pieces that we struggle to tame or make sense of. The dis-order from our dis-ease adds stress when we need it least, and it's natural to blame and question God. *Why is this happening, God? When will it be over? Are you good? Because this doesn't feel good.*

It's perfectly okay to question him, but with our lives resembling a broken puzzle that no longer depicts the beauty it once did, let's remember God is not a God of chaos. His nature, goal, and plans are always to bring peace and order. In the middle of your chaos and questions, take a moment to ask God to encircle you with his peace.

Lord, my life and faith are breaking into pieces. Calm the chaos of my heart and mind. Where I'm confused and questioning, let your peace bring comfort and tranquility. Order the disorder of my disease, fill me with your stillness, and help me see the beauty and harmony of all that you do.

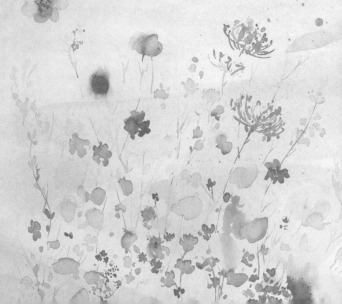

When You're Wrestling
with Faith...

*And Need God's
Provision*

In times of need,

may I need  most.

Safe Inside His Fortress

Turn your ear to me, come quickly to my rescue;
be my rock of refuge, a strong fortress to save me.

PSALM 31:2

Perhaps you need God's provision financially for the mountain of medical bills, or maybe you need his assistance practically in the form of meals, rides for the kids, or someone to put a load of laundry in. The moment we're diagnosed, our needs exponentially escalate, and we're right to ask God for help.

In the midst of the chaos—as the rest of our world, and even our faith, crumbles—let's not forget we also need a safe place to hide: somewhere secure, strong, and impenetrable, containing everything we need. That place is a person: God. He promises to be all these things, so let's pray with confidence because he *will* provide.

Lord, I need your help. Bills are unpaid, the kids need me, and I feel so helpless I want to hide. Hear my cry, Lord, and come quickly. As I shelter in your presence, rescue me. Be my rock, my fortress, and hiding place where I'm safe and sound. I need you, your protection, provision, and peace, now more than ever.

In All Things

*God is able to bless you abundantly, so that in
all things at all times, having all that you need,
you will abound in every good work.*

2 CORINTHIANS 9:8

If you read this verse and assume God's blessing is
conditional on you being fit and healthy enough to
do "good works," like hosting a Bible study or feeding
the homeless, look again. His blessing is actually *so that*
we have all we need in *all things at all times*. Doesn't that
include cancer?

What if, when we're recovering from surgery or
struggling to get out of bed, our good work is simply
to rest and heal? Remember, God is interested in helping you right now, exactly where you are, no matter how
good or bad that is.

*Lord, forgive me for assuming your blessing is contingent
on me showing up for others in ways that right now
sound exhausting. Pour out your blessings in astonishing
ways so I can do the good work of resting, healing, and
recuperating. You're a generous God and know my needs
better than I do, so fill me up until I have all I require.*

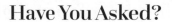

Have You Asked?

Ask and it will be given to you....
For everyone who asks receives.

MATTHEW 7:7-8

How ridiculous would it be to scream at your Starbucks barista for not giving you your coffee order when you never actually asked for it? Crazy, right? Yet we often do the same with God. Sometimes we haven't received simply because we haven't asked. The promise of God is that if we ask, we *will* receive, so if you've asked but feel your pleas have gone unanswered, look around. Maybe they've been answered in unexpected ways, or perhaps what you've received is different from what you prayed for. And if you haven't fully asked, could this be your day to start?

Lord, I'm sorry for getting mad at you for not giving me all I need when I never really take the time to tell you. You promise I'll receive when I ask, so Father, hear my prayers. As I go into my day, open my eyes to the unexpected ways you've already answered. May I, in faith, stand firm on your promise and ask with excited expectation.

The King of the Jungle

The lions may grow weak and hungry,
*but those who seek the L*ORD *lack no good thing.*

PSALM 34:10

I have a huge black-and-white photo of a lion in my living room. He's called Noble. As the king of the jungle, he's strong and courageous, and he never worries where his next meal is coming from. Or that's what I assume. Yet even lions grow tired and hungry at times. We, on the other hand, will lack nothing good when we seek God, and it's not until we seek him that we will find all that is good. On our toughest days, let's look for God before we look for the good stuff.

Today, Lord, I'm going on the hunt. Not for answers to my questions or all the things I need, but for you. Help me pursue you passionately. Grant that when I look for you in every part of my day, I may find you and all I'm looking for. Reassure me of your presence and provision. Remind me daily to seek you first, trusting I have all I need in you.

What Are You Looking For?

*Do not worry....Your heavenly Father knows that you
need them. But seek first his kingdom and his righteousness,
and all these things will be given to you as well.*

MATTHEW 6:31-33

Y ou've got enough to worry about right now. The last
thing you need is to stress over finances, meals, or
your overgrown yard. Thankfully, Jesus tells us the way
to relax, regardless of our needs, is to respond to all God
has already given us—his kingdom and righteousness.
When we immerse ourselves in who God is, what he's
done, and all he gives us, we find our "everyday human
concerns will be met."[13] Take a moment to turn your
gaze from all you need to the one who provides.

*Lord, in my time of greatest need, give me the strength to
shift my attention away from the things I need and want,
focusing it instead on your goodness, love, and generosity.
Help me trust in your unending love for me. Remind me
how I'm more precious to you than the wildflowers, "most
of which are never even seen."[14] May I relax and take
strength from your promise to be here for me, to provide
all I need.*

Blessings, Not Gold Stars

We have confidence before God and receive from him anything we ask, because we keep his commands.

1 JOHN 3:21-22

It's clear there is a connection between our willingness to obey God's commands and his ability to pour out his provision. But let's be careful. It's not because he's a controlling helicopter parent, handing out rewards to ensure his kids do as he says. Far from it. His provision and blessing are a natural consequence of what he asks us to do, not gold stars for completing each task. As you head into chemo, meet with your oncologist, or simply take a needed nap, how might you look to do what pleases God?

Lord, I'm sorry for thinking you're handing out stuff as a reward for good behavior. Remind me of your love for me and how you want what's best for me. Help me keep your commands and do what pleases you simply because I love you, Lord. As I start my day, show me how to walk in obedience, and as I do, may I know and experience your loving provision.

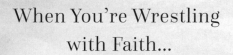

When You're Wrestling
with Faith...

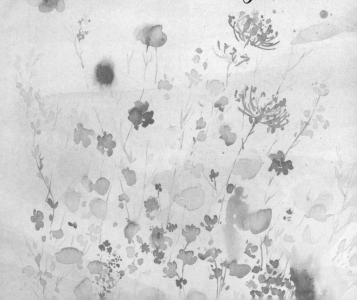

And Asking
for Healing

Make me *well* again, Lord.

A Foundation of Praise

Heal me, Lord, and I will be healed; save me
and I will be saved, for you are the one I praise.

JEREMIAH 17:14

How many times have you begged and pleaded with God for healing? Hundreds probably. And the more we pray and plead, the more desperate and frustrated we become—and the less inclined we are to praise him. Unlike Jeremiah, who praises God while he's sick, suffering, and praying for healing, we hold our praises until we see our Creator move.

Take a moment to give thanks to God in the midst of your illness, not just when he heals. Make praise the foundation of your prayers for healing, and worship God for who he is.

Lord, you are the one I praise. Forgive me for coming to you in anger and frustration. Today I come in praise and thanksgiving for who you are. You are my everything, and I worship you. In sickness and in health, I give you my trust and my life because you are my God. You are mighty to save, and so I pray, "Heal me, Lord, and I will be healed; save me and I will be saved. For you are the one I praise."

His Way, His Time

*The prayer offered in faith will make the
sick person well; the Lord will raise them up.*

JAMES 5:15

If this verse has ever been used to suggest God hasn't
healed you because you don't have enough faith, I'm
so sorry. In Scripture, faith and healing are always con-
nected, but there's no vending machine where we can
put faith in, push the prayer button, and out comes
healing. There's mystery involved—and so much we
don't know. One thing we do know, however, is we only
need a mustard seed's worth of faith. True, genuine
faith, even a speck as tiny as the seed of a mustard plant,
acknowledges that Jesus *will* heal in his way and in his
time. Let's place our trust and faith—no matter how
miniscule, no matter how frail—in Jesus today.

*Lord, my faith is small and weak, but what I have is true
and genuine. Help me trust your will and your ways, and
as I do, would you heal my cancer? Lord, shrink the tumor
inside me, remove any cancer cells seeking new places to
grow in my body, and restore me to full health. Set me on
my feet again. Raise me up, Lord.*

Seen and Heard

This is what the LORD, the God of your
father David, says: I have heard your prayer
and seen your tears; I will heal you.

2 KINGS 20:5

I remember as a kid standing on a cliff, shouting, "Hello there" into the distance before hearing the lonely echo return to me. I wondered, *Did my words come back because there was no one to hear them and no place to land?*

Sweet friend, the ocean of tears you've cried and the innumerable prayers you've prayed haven't echoed off the heavens unseen and unheard. Trust me, even prayers seemingly met with silence and inaction are heard and seen. So let's wait with expectation.

Weeping into the night and crying into the silence, I've felt so alone and unseen, Lord. But I'm not. You witness every tear as it falls to the ground. You catch every prayer as it echoes into the darkness. Yes, Lord, I want healing right this minute—yesterday, if I'm honest—but I wait with hope and prayerful expectation that you, the God of David, the God who has been faithful forever, the God who hears and sees me, will also heal me.

He Understands

By his wounds you have been healed.

1 PETER 2:24

As our blood counts remain stubbornly elevated or our tumors continue to light up a PET scan like a Christmas tree, it's confusing and hard to hear that at some level, we've already been healed. Yet it's true. Jesus suffered and died a painful death to restore us to life in his Father, and it's because of the wounds he endured that we can be confident he both understands our suffering and continues to work for our ongoing healing and restoration.

Thank you, Jesus!

Knowing you understand what it's like to go through something painful and terrifying comforts me, Jesus. It renews my faith as I battle on, continually praying for healing as I go. By your wounds I'm healed, so today I ask, in your precious name, that you heal my body just as your Father healed yours. May all you did on the cross restore me to full health in the same way it restored me to a full relationship with you.

We Have the Power

He gave them power and authority to
drive out all demons and to cure diseases.

LUKE 9:1

Jesus didn't leave the question of whether his disciples should pray for the sick open to debate. He repeatedly told them they had power and authority to pray, deal with demons, and cure diseases, and he expected them to walk in that power.

Amazingly, he continues today to give that same strength and influence to you, me, and your Christian friends—to pray in his name. Asking others to pray for us and with us can be hard, yet as disciples, we have his power and authority to do so.

Who could you ask to pray for you today in his power and authority?

Jesus, help me walk through this cancer and pray for healing with your power and authority. Forgive me for forgetting how much command over sickness and the enemy you've given me. As I ask friends to pray in your powerful name, would you pour out that authority and healing? You are the God of miracles, Lord. May we see your miraculous healing today.

Reaching Out in Faith

He said to her, "Daughter, your faith has healed you.
Go in peace and be freed from your suffering."

MARK 5:34

It had been twelve difficult years, and after "a long succession of physicians had treated her, and treated her badly, taking all her money and leaving her worse off than before,"[15] her goal was simply to touch Jesus's cloak. Believing this one act could make her well, she pushed through the crowd, stretched out her hand, brushed her fingers against his robe, and left the rest in God's hands. Whether you've been battling cancer for twelve days or twelve years, can you follow in this courageous woman's footsteps? Take a moment to reach out to Jesus in faith, trusting him with your healing.

Lord, sometimes I don't have the strength or determination to push through the crowds to get to you, or the faith to believe simply touching you will heal me. Increase my trust in you. Help me weave through the many doctors, appointments, and worries jostling me from every side. Help me connect with you in faith. I believe you can make me well. Heal me, Lord.

When You're Wrestling
with Faith...

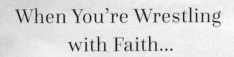

But Still Want
to Praise God

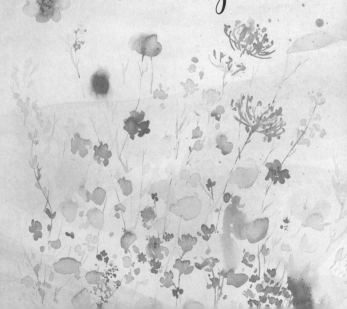

Through aching and weeping,

may my *praises*

never grow silent.

Go for It

You turned my wailing into dancing...
that my heart may sing your praises and not be silent.

PSALM 30:11-12

At some point in every cancer journey God does something amazing. Even in the middle of our questioning, heaviness, and wrestling, he finds ways to break through and do something marvelous. If that's happened, don't hold it in. Allow your cries of anguish and exhaustion to become feet-tapping, arm-raising praise. Go for it. As you worship and give thanks for what he has done, other worries and questions will begin to fade.

When God turns things around, even for a minute, let's transform our worry into worship.

Even in the midst of my doubts, frustration, and wrestling, you show up in unbelievable ways, letting me know that I am deeply cherished, that I am fully seen. O Lord, how mighty and loving you are! I can't hold it in or be silent. When my worries and weeping overtake me, help me remember your goodness and glorify you anyway. You're simply the best, Lord, and I shout your praises.

The Catalyst

About midnight Paul and Silas were
praying and singing hymns to God....
Suddenly there was such a violent earthquake.

ACTS 16:25-26

It's dark and damp in the prison, but as they sit—chained, forgotten, and with little hope of release—Paul and Silas don't grumble, lose hope, or rant at God about how unfair life is. They pray and worship.

Praise erupts from deep within us when God breaks into our pain, doing something miraculous, but it's rarely our go-to response when we feel trapped and afraid. Yet in the Bible worship is often the catalyst to breakthrough. As Paul and Silas worshipped, the prison doors flew open, and the invitation to us is the same: to lift our hearts in worship no matter where we are, placing ourselves in the hands of the God of breakthrough.

You are the God of miracles and the God of breakthroughs. I worship and praise you from the darkness of my cancer prison. Lord, whether your mighty hand stretches out to release me or not, I will sing of your goodness and pray for your presence. Fling wide the doors, Lord!

The Door to Praise

*Enter his gates with thanksgiving
and his courts with praise; give thanks
to him and praise his name.*

PSALM 100:4

My kids hated writing thank-you notes. Yet once they'd penned a few lines about how they'd built their new Lego set or twirled for hours in their sparkly princess costume, they ended up loving not just their gift but the gift-giver even more.

In the same way, when we thank God, we see who he is and what he has given us more clearly. Our love and adoration for him grow. Gratitude opens the door to praise, drawing us into his presence. This is why the simple act of giving thanks is such a powerful spiritual discipline.

Let's enter his courts today with our thank-you notes raised high.

Here, from the midst of my cancer—and, if I'm honest, with a heart that's not always grateful—I want to thank you, Lord. I often forget to thank you for simply being you. You are more wonderful than I can pen words to express. You love me deeper than I can truly comprehend. Even when life isn't good, you are. I praise you, Lord.

Bubbling Within You

I waited patiently for the LORD.... He set
my feet on a rock.... He put a new song in
my mouth, a hymn of praise to our God.

PSALM 40:1-3

Hurry up and wait." It's the familiar refrain to our cancer melody. We're rushed into testing or surgery, and then we wait endlessly for results or for our bodies to heal. It's one of the worst things about having cancer. Worrying and waiting are tortuous.

Yet when we wait for God to see us, show up, or hear our cries—which he always does—he plants our feet on solid ground and shows us more of who he is. From here come new songs of praise.

What is the new song he's caused to bubble up within you?

Lord, I've waited for you through endless nights and tear-filled days, and you saw me and heard me. I'm no longer being tossed around by my cancer but am on solid ground where I won't lose my footing, so I give you glory. Even though I can't hold a tune, I sing praises to your name. In the weeks and months ahead, help me remember this truth and teach me to always hurry and wait for you.

The One He Wants

Ascribe to the LORD the glory due his name;
bring an offering and come before him.

1 CHRONICLES 16:29

I wonder if the shepherd who brought baby Jesus the gift of a lamb felt his offering was too small and inadequate? After all, shepherds and sheep were far from special in Bethlehem. In the same way, it's easy to think we have nothing to offer to the Lord.

We don't have huge wealth or a gift for evangelism to rival Billy Graham, and what we do have—a body deteriorating from cancer—can leave us feeling like our gifts, possessions, or even good works are woefully pitiful. Thankfully, God simply wants our hearts.

As you worship God today, don't just "ascribe to him the glory due his name" but also bring the one offering he really desires—you.

Lord, I know it's not much, but I bring you all I've got: me. As an act of worship, praise, and gratitude, I give you my heart in all its wounded brokenness. You are worthy of anything and everything I can give you, so I come to you today offering the praise and glory due your name. I am yours. Help me give you more of me.

Sing Out

Though the fig tree does not bud and there are no grapes on the vines...yet I will rejoice in the LORD.

HABAKKUK 3:17-18

Life with or without cancer can be a roller coaster of highs and lows. One minute everything is going swimmingly, and the next we're drowning, struggling to catch a breath.

Whether you're on top of the world or watching your world crumble, you're invited to rejoice and glory in the one who never changes. In him there's much to sing about.

No matter where we are, let's praise God.

Today, focus on Jesus. Take joy in who he is, knowing he loves you, is with you, and has your life in the palm of his hands.

Lord, even though I look around and everything in my life seems barren, broken, or burned, I will rejoice, delighting in your love for me. You are the God who holds me, whose plans are good, and who will never leave. May I never forget you are the one who has conquered all, the one who is mighty and merciful. How can I not rejoice and be glad? How can I not give thanks for your goodness?

When You're Wrestling
with Faith...

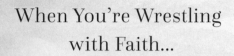

*And Not Feeling
Good Enough for God*

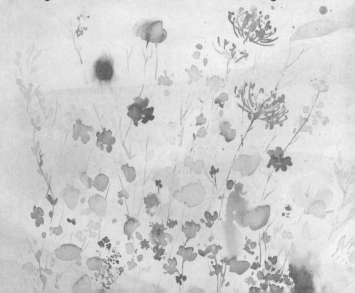

In my imperfections,
may I rest in your
perfect grace.

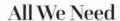

All We Need

He said to me, "My grace is sufficient for you,
for my power is made perfect in weakness."

2 CORINTHIANS 12:9

I admit it. I'm a "hold it all together at all costs" kind of girl who likes to appear strong and unfazed by life's struggles. I don't remember being told weakness equals inadequacy, but somehow the message burrowed deeply: Weak meant unlovable.

We may wear strength outwardly to ensure we're loved, but God is fully aware of our weaknesses, and if we're willing to bring them to Jesus, we discover his infinite grace. His love isn't based on who or what we are but on who and what he is— love—so we can drop our show of strength. His grace is all we need.

Will you risk being real before him today?

Lord, I feel so inadequate and I just hate it. I want to come to you strong and on top of things. But I'm not. Help me be real with you, and in my weakness, show me your grace and love. When I shy away from you, assuming you'll reject me because I'm not good enough, remind me you love me as I am.

Just as You Are

Blessed are the meek, for they will inherit the earth.

MATTHEW 5:5

If you worry about being good enough for God, you're probably closer to him than you think! In the kingdom of God, meekness is a virtue. When people know they're not top dog or the bee's knees and come to God just as they are, they are blessed. These folks will inherit the earth.

If that's you, can you turn your fears into prayers? Come to him as your real, honest self, not the person you think you should be. You'll not only inherit the earth but be "inwardly peaceful, spiritually secure."[16]

Doesn't that sound wonderful?

Lord, I don't have to earn your love, peace, or blessing, but when it comes to this truth, I have the receptivity of a rhino and the memory of a goldfish. May my fears and failures be offerings of honesty. As I come to you with every mess-up, doubt, question, and inadequacy on full show, would you bring the peace and security I can only find in you?

Heavenly Etiquette

*Let us then approach God's throne of grace
with confidence, so that we may receive mercy
and find grace to help us in our time of need.*

HEBREWS 4:16

I'm a Brit, and although my knowledge of royal court etiquette is limited, I do know you can't just waltz up to the throne whenever you fancy. There are rules and protocols. You need an invitation to approach Her Majesty. Thankfully, it's the opposite with God. There is no bowing or scraping, no waiting to be summoned, and absolutely no checks to ensure we're doing, saying, or wearing the right thing. His throne is a place of grace. Everyone is welcome, and it's where we find the help we need.

You can't walk right up to the Queen, but there is nothing stopping you from approaching God's throne of grace in prayer today.

Lord, I'm grateful I don't have to jump through a thousand hoops or be on my best behavior to enter your presence. I need your mercy, help, and grace, so I come to you just as I am. Fill me with them afresh. Show me how loved I am. Remind me how welcome I am in your presence.

With You Always

Surely I am with you always, to the very end of the age.

MATTHEW 28:20

The disciples were a hot mess. They fought amongst themselves, fell asleep when Jesus needed them most, and professed undying devotion before denying him. Yet Jesus loved them.

Knowing they'd mess up, face trials, and struggle in their faith, he still found them worthy of purpose, sending them out into the world to carry on his work, and his promise to them—to be by their side through it all, always—is for us too.

No matter how messed up we are, what we have or haven't done, or how insecure or inadequate we feel, he is with us. He is with *you*, dear friend—right here, right now.

I'm flawed, full of doubts, and feeling wholly insufficient for you, Lord. Remind me of your love. Remind me how you'll never leave me, ever. As I head into the cancer world, comfort and encourage me with your presence and reassure me there is nothing I can't face with you beside me.

The New You

If anyone is in Christ, the new creation has come:
The old has gone, the new is here!

2 CORINTHIANS 5:17

The past is a great place to visit, but it's a terrible place to set up camp. Too often we find ourselves burning with regret, churning every terrible decision, or stuck in the paralyzing hurt inflicted by someone's unkind words or abusive actions. We hang out in the *old*, forgetting we've been made *new*.

As Christians, we get a fresh start, but too often we hang out in our old self and assume God will reject its ugliness. To Jesus you're a new creation, pure and holy in him. Can you see yourself that way as well?

It's hard to believe you see me as something new, beautiful, and holy. A fresh creation. Forgive me for clinging to the old me and thinking that's the person you see and will ultimately reject. Today I choose to see myself as you do. May I walk in the reality of being made new in you. As the old fades, may the belief I'm not good enough vanish with it. The old me has gone. I am new!

Grace Guaranteed

You then... be strong in the grace that is in Christ Jesus.

2 TIMOTHY 2:1

Weapons empower armies and profits build up businesses, but neither are guaranteed. We, on the other hand, are strong in grace: a grace that's 100 percent guaranteed and will never fade or be snatched away. We will always have access to the love of God.

I don't know about you, but I find such relief in this. When my faith and self-worth hit rock bottom, when I feel totally unlovable, I soothe and strengthen my aching soul with this reminder: God's love is wholly based on who he is, not who I am.

Take a moment to allow his grace to strengthen you.

Thank you for your grace, Lord God. You love me without limits or conditions—even when I struggle to love myself and find nothing of value within me. Cancer has stolen so much of my strength—physical, emotional, and especially spiritual—so in my doubts and weakness, may your grace fortify me, encourage me, and bring fresh relief to my weary, worried soul. Give me strength, through your grace, to face whatever comes my way.

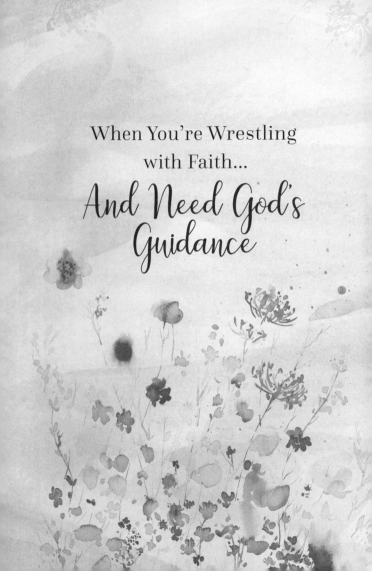

When You're Wrestling
with Faith...
And Need God's Guidance

May your *guidance* be clear and my willingness to follow, bold.

Figuring It Out Together

*If any of you lacks wisdom, you should
ask God...and it will be given to you.*

JAMES 1:5

If we need wisdom, we just need to ask God. It sounds simple, and yet how often do we actually ask him? We happily ask friends, family, doctors, pastors, and even our hairdresser for advice, so why not God? Often, we simply don't think to ask him—or it's a last resort when we've exhausted all other options.

As a mom, I love it when my kids come to me for guidance. I try not to fix things for them but listen and help them figure it out for themselves. God is the same. He wants to help us figure it out.

Let's bring him our confusions and questions today, confident that when we do, he'll pour out his promised wisdom upon us.

Lord, it's good to be reminded of this promise. So often I struggle with what to do, and I hate to admit it, but asking you isn't on my radar. Forgive me for struggling on alone. I need your wisdom and guidance today. Show me a way through, one that I couldn't see alone, and help me figure this out.

Our Ultimate Cancer Guide

When he, the Spirit of truth, comes,
he will guide you into all the truth.

JOHN 16:13

My husband is a great tour guide. Before we visit anywhere, he researches a place's history and the best spots to eat and explore, so we rarely get lost or spend half a day figuring out what to do next. It's wonderfully stress-free.

Maybe you have a cancer "tour guide." I did. Her name was Darcy, and as my cancer navigator, she helped guide me through my disease. I loved her, but our ultimate life-guide and cancer navigator will always be the Holy Spirit.

The Spirit of God can do so much: guide you through the confusion and stress of life with cancer, show you the way, help you understand what's going on and what decisions to make. He will stop you from getting lost.

The question is, will you let him?

Lord, I'm lost and confused and don't know what to do next. Take my hand. Be my guide. Help me make sense of what has happened, show me which way to go, and give me the light to see a way forward. Fill me with your guiding Spirit, O Lord, and lead me always to what is true.

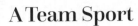

A Team Sport

*The way of fools seems right to them,
but the wise listen to advice.*

PROVERBS 12:15

I hate to admit it, but when I was first diagnosed, I didn't want anything to do with the cancer community. Determined to survive, I hunkered down with my stiff upper lip firmly in place—until surviving was all I was doing. Eventually I discovered that thriving is a team sport: No one wins alone.

You could rely on yourself like I did, but it's so much better to have people who can be God's hands, feet, and voice in your life to love, encourage, and guide you.

Take a moment to ask God to bring the right people into your life and to help you seek the love and guidance you need.

Lord, sometimes the reason I don't know what to do next is because I've shut everyone out, including you. I'm sorry for going it alone and not listening to others. I just don't find it easy. Surround me with people who'll speak into my life and help me ask for and receive the love and advice I so desperately need. Open my heart and ears to others, Lord.

Asking Afraid

Search me, God, and know my heart;
test me and know my anxious thoughts....
And lead me in the way everlasting.

PSALM 139:23-24

I often try to get my fears in check before I ask God for guidance. Unfortunately, it means fear, not faith, drives my actions. Not so for King David. Freely admitting his mind is racing with anxiety, he calls on God to thoroughly dive into his thoughts. Only then does he ask God to lead him. His faith, not his fear, led the way.

Today, can you move ahead in faith, not fear, allowing the Spirit to search your heart and see your anxious mind *before* you ask for guidance? Doing so always leads to freedom or, as King David says, the way everlasting.

Jesus, search my heart and know my every hidden fear. Praying this feels scary, but no matter what you find, I know your love is unchanging. Help me step forward in faith, not fear. Show me the way—the way that always leads back to you and the freedom found in you—the way everlasting. Faith, not fear. Your way, not mine.

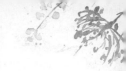

Your Choice

*Be very careful, then, how you live....Do not
be foolish, but understand what the Lord's will is.*

EPHESIANS 5:15-17

In the thick of my treatment, every decision seemed to be made by someone else, from when I was to have scans, chemo, and surgery to what drugs pumped through my veins—and, yes, even how I'd poop (hello, ostomy bag!). Yet every day, no matter what I faced, I did have a choice: to live "foolishly" or seek to follow the Lord's will.

Whatever you're up to today, as you try and figure out your next step, ask yourself these two questions: What is God saying? Am I willing to do it?

Lord, you know how foolish and thoughtless I've been. Not only have I failed to understand what your will is, but I didn't even ask what it might be in the first place. Oh, forgive me. Help me make the decisions I need to make. But more than that, show me how to make the most of my life and not waste it. When I don't seek your will or do as you prompt, my life fritters away, so tell me what you want of me, Lord. I will do it.

Sweet Relief

The LORD will guide you always;
he will satisfy your needs in a sun-scorched land
and will strengthen your frame.

ISAIAH 58:11

I t doesn't *always* rain in England, but as a Brit transplanted to the heat and humidity of the Carolinas, I've never quite acclimatized. During the summer of my cancer treatment, as the roads shimmered with heat haze, and the sun-scorched, cancer-filled days reduced me to a weak, lethargic, air-conditioning-loving mess, this verse brought sweet relief physically, as well as spiritually.

God promises to show us the way and, as he does, to satiate our longings and strengthen our withering bodies. What a blessing! What better reason to seek his guidance today in the middle of your cancer-scorched life?

I'm withering and wilting in the sun-scorched wasteland of my cancer, Lord, and I don't know which way to turn. My body aches. It cries out for your guidance and strength. As my heart yearns for your love, my feet long to step where you lead. Show me the way. Rebuild my broken life into the full life you have for me. Strengthen me in my weakness.

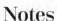

Notes

1. Saint Augustine, *Confessions*, book 3, paragraph 11.

2. Pete Greig, *How to Pray: A Simple Guide for Normal People* (Colorado Springs, CO: NavPress, 2019).

3. Psalm 30:5 MSG.

4. Psalm 56:8 ESV.

5. Alfred, Lord Tennyson, *The Higher Pantheism*, https://www.poetry foundation.org/poems/45323/the-higher-pantheism.

6. Habakkuk 2:3 MSG.

7. Romans 8:28 MSG.

8. This phrase is from Elisabeth Elliot, *Suffering Is Never for Nothing* (Nashville, TN: B&H, 2019).

9. 1 Corinthians 16:13 MSG.

10. Jeremiah 29:11 MSG.

11. Adapted from Romans 12:1 MSG.

12. Jeremiah 33:3 MSG.

13. Matthew 6:33 MSG.

14. Matthew 6:30 MSG.

15. Mark 5:29 MSG.

16. Matthew 5:5 AMP.

About the Author

Niki Hardy is an author, speaker, podcast host, and cancer thriver.

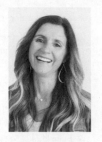

Through her books, including *Break Free from Survival Mode: 7 Ways to Thrive Through Hard Times,* her down-to-earth devotional-style podcast, *Chemo Chair Prayers,* and her Trusting God Through Cancer Summit, Niki wants to help you discover life doesn't have to be pain-free to be full, then show you how to live it.

When she's not writing or speaking, you can find her walking her two lovely but rather stupid Goldendoodles, or trying to figure out which remote actually turns the TV on.

Learn more and find FREE resources at
www.nikihardy.com
Follow her on Instagram @niki.hardy

More from Niki Hardy

Register for her FREE
Trusting God Through Cancer Summit
www.trustinggodthroughcancer.com

* * *

Listen to her podcast
www.chemochairprayers.com